SURPRISED
BY
NOTHING

SURPRISED BY NOTHING

Surviving the ER World of Worst-Case Scenarios

Kathryn Kyker

GFB

Published by GFB™, Seattle
www.girlfridayproductions.com

Produced by Girl Friday Productions

Cover design: Emily Weigel
Production editorial: Katherine Richards
Project management: Abi Pollokoff

Image credits: cover © Shutterstock/JACKREZNOR

ISBN (hardcover): 978-1-964721-61-3
ISBN (paperback): 978-1-964721-60-6
ISBN (ebook): 978-1-964721-59-0

Library of Congress Control Number: 2025912843

First edition

To the patients and families I met in their worst moments,
and to the health care team
that works bravely in those hard places:
All of you were my teachers
and my constant companions in this writing and remembering.

When we stop distancing ourselves from the pain in the world, our own or others', we create the possibility of a new experience, one that often surprises because of how much joy, connection, or relief it yields. Destruction may continue, but humanity shines through.

—Mark Epstein, *The Trauma of Everyday Life*

Contents

IMAGINE

ACT

LISTEN

Preface

"You love your stories." This is what the computer analyst at the hospital said to me as we reviewed the new charting system. We were making the transition from paper to electronic documentation. The analyst had once worked in the ER and was familiar with all the roles in the department. He wanted to create drop-down lists and checkboxes to categorize our interventions with patients. But from the social work perspective, every patient's set of circumstances was unique, and while medicine seeks to find commonality—a diagnosis label expedites treatment—effective social work depends on awareness of unique differences. He gave us some open text boxes instead—room for us to write stories.

Our stories say what we did for a patient and include relevant dynamics, a sort of code for the next social worker: *Patient acknowledged that she knew the alleged abuser* is code for possible domestic violence. *Patient and mother demonstrated attachment as mother comforted her* lets me know that a social worker was involved, but a report of abuse or neglect was not needed. *Patient declined referral* tells me our offer of assistance was rejected. Such nuanced notations are essential for painting a picture of the visit.

Writing the story inside the chart, paper or electronic, is challenging. Sharing our stories outside the ER is formidable. Bound by professional ethics and hospital confidentiality, we can relate stories only in the most general and nonidentifying way.

My story converged with many others': patients, their families, my coworkers and administrators, my family. My intention is to share only what is essential. Patient names and incident details have all been changed in numerous ways. My first professional supervisor said, "The mark of a good social worker is a well-bitten tongue." I hope I've bit mine the right amount.

When people learn I worked in an ER, they often ask me to relate the "craziest thing you saw." In order to tell an entertaining story while avoiding identifying details, I have to put myself in the place of the audience and emphasize the funniest or most dramatic bits. But those bits are always tangled up in a larger, sadder story. Not including *those* bits feels like a betrayal—to the patient, to myself, and to a larger truth.

Foreign objects stuck in body cavities seem funny enough unless you recall the patient was burdened by a history of such acts, a compulsive behavior causing harm and humiliation. I once greeted a mom with the news that her adult child just had a colostomy but couldn't say it was due to sexual play with kitchen utensils. I can think of no crazy stories that are not stained with sorrow.

When I'm asked to "tell the craziest thing," I don't. I try to avoid an awkward pause. I give them a look designed to make them feel that they already know the answer, as if I am bringing them into my secret reality. My head tilts. "It's pretty crazy," I say. Then I pivot to a question about them.

The truth is that person doesn't really want to hear those stories, at least not in the way I would tell them. They don't make for good small talk. I want to tell the deeper story—how I have been affected by what happened to strangers. The stories I share are the ones I claim because they have claimed me. They had an impact on my life, became embedded in my mind and my body. The need to understand my experience through sharing it has finally overcome all the inherent obstacles and fears. And though my experience is unique, I believe what I've learned about my personal response to stress and trauma is relevant to most of us, no matter where or if you work. I explore the challenges of providing help, professionally and personally, through the length of my career and into retirement, and the cost of being driven to make a difference.

My time in the ER flipped my reality and scrambled my sense of security, but I do not blame the hospital, the staff and providers, or medical systems for whatever issues, thoughts, or behaviors I ended up with when my time there was over. I know that I came in with certain tendencies and challenges that shaped the effects of my ER experiences. Did having an "overactive imagination" (as my mother puts it) make the gritty truth of an ER shift more visceral? Did my tendency toward storymaking facilitate or complicate my work as a patient advocate and then manager?

I use the titles "ER social worker" and "patient advocate" interchangeably. I am a professional social worker and identified myself as such in the ER. However, a social work degree was not required for the position I initially worked in and later supervised, and the term *advocate* may be more descriptive of the role. Most professional social workers in hospitals work with admitted patients and do a very different sort of work.

We called it the "ER" back then, but years later the term got changed to ED—Emergency Department—because, of course, it is an entire department. I refer to it as the ER out of sentiment, as a nod to my beginnings, and because it sounds way cooler.

I worked in only one ER, but I generalize my observations. I benefited from the experiences of my coworkers and directors, who worked in a variety of ERs, and attended conferences to glean knowledge of how others succeeded or failed. I know each ER is different. What was true for "my" ER may not be true for others. My examples may paint nurses or doctors in a certain shade, but they are all over the spectrum. I find fault with the ER and our medical system in general, and I offer no solutions.

The ER is a dumping station, a continual come-as-you-are party, and ground zero for our nation's health care crisis. It's no surprise that it's a flawed place full of terrors. It's a toxic mix of near disasters and insufficient resources. There's no reason to expect so much good to come out of the ER so often, but it does. An ER can be the best example of modern alchemy—miracles are rare, but transformation does happen, and in real time and by ordinary mortals.

This could be a story about . . .

- our health care system
- how I hid my fear of blood
- how I raised my children in the shadow of every horrible thing possible
- how imagination is both my superpower and my kryptonite
- how I lost the ability to cry
- how listening always helps
- why superstition works
- how I used detachment as a survival skill
- how caring for a living meant I didn't have to care so much on my own time
- how I no longer believe that things happen for a reason
- how most people are more decent than you should ever expect.

It is a story about every one of those things.

I worked in an ER from age twenty-eight to fifty-seven. I came in as one person and left as another.

I like to think that the ER changed too, that my time there made it better in some small way, but the ER sheds without sentiment anything that no longer works or has become too much trouble in the eyes of whoever calls the shots. If I left anything lasting there, it was only the impression that I, or my work, made on the people I met.

Those impressions may have been positive, but they were created by a woman in denial of the price she paid. My inability to clearly see this in the moment makes me question my intuition. I am an unreliable narrator. My perspective is flawed, yet it is my only guide through this experience.

If you picked up this book because you harbor an inclination to work in an ER, I hope you retain that desire after reading it, because the ER needs you, and not many people are up to it. Just know the snake you pick up: The ER is part of a broken system. It does not change quickly, yet it never stays the same. It will reveal secrets about your community you will never forget. It will introduce you to the smell of a GI bleed and the feel of a dead body. It will not cure many of its patients. Working there will not cure your inner wounds. You will learn to laugh in the dark, but no one outside the ER will understand your laughter.

The League of Blood and Guts

DFO: Done Fell Out, as in, *"We were in Walmart. She seemed fine, but then all of a sudden, she done fell out."* As used by medics in the South: *"We're bringing in a woman who DFO'ed in Walmart."*

The medical term for falling out is *syncope*. Symptoms include lightheadedness and sometimes tunnel vision. I also get cold sweats and heart palpitations. I've fallen out twice. The first time, I was a teenager sleeping over at a friend's house. We were in the bathroom, washing our faces with the diligence of acne-prone adolescents. She wanted to tell me about a show she'd seen about eye surgery—in all its gory detail.

She mimed how they cut into the eye and pulled back the layers. I got swimmy. I told her to stop. I knew this feeling because I had almost fainted in third grade when the teacher explained why blood is red.

My friend ignored my protest. She persisted in explaining the surgical procedure. When I came to, I was on the floor, my foot kicking the space heater. My friend knelt beside me, tearfully spouting apologies. She thought she'd killed me.

I knew I was squeamish, the label affixed to me by a school nurse back in third grade. My mom chalked it up to my "vivid imagination" (which wasn't a compliment).

My vivid imagination was the reason that I could not eat cauliflower once I saw it whole, because it looked like a brain; why I still can't eat dates, because they look like roaches; why I went to the dictionary at age ten to look up the ingredients in food that jiggled—and discovered what gelatin is. As an adult, I am, of course, a pescatarian. I don't cook fish, but I'll eat it as long as it isn't presented to me with intact eyeballs.

Like a mischievous friend, my imagination could get me into trouble, but it was also a faithful companion that eased loneliness, provided comfort, and gave me a sense of power. It led me to get lost in complex fantasies that required time alone—on my swing set, hiding under the stairs, ambling around the neighborhood—when I was supposed to be folding clothes or emptying the dishwasher. My parents blamed my imagination for my nightmares, for my storytelling (my family called this "lying"), and for that near-fainting incident in third grade.

The second time I fell out was right in front of Mom. I was an undergraduate student studying social work, home from college during a break, and we were watching a horror movie. When a werewolf tore into a victim's throat, I got up to leave the room. I came to on the floor, my mom leaning over me. She wasn't freaked out. She had the put-upon, "I told you so" look that comes so naturally to a mother—passing out was my punishment for failing to get that imagination under control.

About ten years after that incident, the ER hired me as a patient advocate. I hadn't DFO'ed in all that time, but of course my mother hadn't forgotten. When I told her about my new job, she busted out laughing.

"Do they know you're afraid of blood?" She couldn't imagine this new job working out.

I wasn't trying to prove anything; I just needed the job. My husband and I were trying to save money to move out of a rental house and buy a home close to a good school. He was working overtime. I was a contract worker for the adoption agency where I did my internship for my master's degree. My work was part-time, and as the economy dipped, the number of families choosing to pursue adoption slowed to a trickle. The next year our son would start kindergarten. We needed to move right away; I needed to earn more money.

I had bumped into a social worker friend who was leaving her part-time job in the ER. She told me what the job entailed—it was a good fit for a social worker's skill set.

Shift work was appealing. I could manage a few shifts around my other job and limit the amount of childcare we needed. My friend promised the job would offer a variety of patients and tasks, and almost no paperwork—a rarity in the field of social work. I was sold. By the time I had the interview I was almost positive I could handle it.

The director of the ER had a low-lit, homey office. There were pictures of her family on her desk, and her children's drawings decorated the walls. I could almost smell cookies baking. Her desk was pushed against a wall, such that she and I sat side by side, instead of a desk blocking the space between us. This impressed me. Desk placement is my litmus test for gauging how secure a boss is in their authority.

As her interest in me as a candidate became apparent, I confessed my DFO issue. She assured me that the blood and guts were for the medical professionals. I wouldn't have to concern myself with anything I couldn't handle. I believed her. She offered the job, and I took it.

Horror movie images aside, in real life, I discovered that I'm not afraid of the sight of blood generally. Bloody wounds, gaping holes, spurting blood? Not really a problem. I can wipe up a trail of blood that follows a gurney down the hallway and sop up blood that pools into eyelids from a head wound. I can even hold a child down as an IV is started, as long as I stare at the wall while they insert the needle. But blood in tubes, blood in bags, and blood being filtered by dialysis—*contained* blood—was a problem.

This is not to say that more graphic displays of free-flowing blood and guts do not get to me. Torn skin is disturbing, as are burns. Fractures, with their unnatural contortions, make my gut flip, and chronic wounds elicit revulsion and empathy via smell even if I don't see them. But I'd rather be in a room with any of those patients than the one placidly receiving blood.

You'd think I would have known better than to try donating blood, but I did not. As a college student I gave blood a few times. Turns out I am an "easy stick" (good veins). My heart is willing, but my blood flow is reluctant. It always took me longer to fill up the clear plastic pouch than anyone around me. Donors came and went while I struggled on, eyes shut tight to avoid seeing all that blood contained. When my body had finally relinquished 460 mL, I had a lengthy enforced detention at the snack table. I tried repeatedly to stand and walk away, but only wobbled. The nurses kept wrangling me back, pushing juice and cookies. The third time I donated blood the nurse excused me from ever coming back. I was probably blowing their budget for snacks.

Just as with that third-grade lecture and my friend's description of eye surgery, certain conversations still bothered me. Eating in the small ER staff break room subjected me to shoptalk, as the nurses, techs, and sometimes doctors reviewed cases and procedures, eager to share and learn from each other. I persisted and over time achieved a measure of desensitization. Occasionally I still did have to ask for a change of subject. My coworkers were always kind about that, quickly remembering that I was not part of their blood-and-guts league. We worked in the same place, took care of the same patients, but in very different ways. They knew that outside the ER, their fascination was considered grotesque for the dinner table.

The people of medicine are a different sort of people. They say, "We didn't kill anyone today," to mark a good shift. They are intrigued by situations that make the rest of us feel aversion. If I had fallen out in front of my coworkers, they would have taken care of me. But once I was back on my feet, the teasing that followed would have been hell, and the story would be passed along and handed down to dog me all my days.

I knew that if any of them witnessed me passing out, they'd never stop watching me. I'd see a look gleaming with amused curiosity and the unspoken inquiry: *"Are you gonna DFO?"* They would know my "squeamish buttons" and could even use them against me. I would be less of an asset and more of a liability, a distraction, or, worse, entertainment. I resolved never to hit the floor in the ER.

A therapist once told me that the key to not passing out is to know you are not trapped once the symptoms start. I usually employed this strategy with success, but it failed me once when I was escorting a family to a patient's room. They got into a discussion of some element of the patient's medical issue that bothered me. I tried stepping away, tried to lead them forward, tried to interrupt the conversation, but nothing worked. They were glued in place as they went deeper into gory descriptions, and I was thrust further and further down that narrowing tunnel.

Finally, I walked to a nearby chair, sat, and stated I didn't feel well. They immediately stopped talking, turning their attention to me. They assumed I was pregnant. And I let them.

This has happened less as time's gone on, though movies can still be a challenge. I had to walk out of both *Interview with the Vampire* and *Black Swan*. Fortunately, I never encountered a ballet-dancing vampire in the ER, nor met any of my coworkers in the cinema bathroom as I sat on the floor, back against the wall, head between my knees—an imposter in the League of Blood and Guts.

The Rule of Three

You know this rule. You see it in movies when the heroine takes aim at the charging monster. She misses once, then twice—she's almost done for!—but the third time's the charm. The failed attempts ratchet up the stakes and suspense, we feel her desperation, then we're granted a delicious relief.

There's a limit to how much unsuccessful striving an audience wants to see. Three attempts is the magic number. As audiences grow wise to such techniques, some writers subvert expectations by breaking this rule. Expectations sabotaged can evoke more delight than expectations met. But to break a rule it must first exist.

The hero's journey, popularized by Joseph Campbell and adapted into a writer's guide by Christopher Vogler, has three main parts: the preparation or call to the journey, the journey itself, and the return home.[1]

The structure survives because audiences find it satisfying, perhaps because we think of our external lives in three parts: youth, adulthood, and old age. For our internal life, Freud proposed we have the id, ego, and superego. Jung proposed a different three: ego, personal unconscious, and collective unconscious, or more basically, ego, self, and soul.[2]

I, too, seek a rule of three to orient and anchor me.

---

1. Joseph Campbell with Bill Moyers, *The Power of Myth* (Doubleday, 1988); Christopher Vogler, *The Writer's Journey* (Michael Wiese Productions, 2007).
2. Ernest M. Oleksy, "A Brief Review of Freudian and Jungian Theories," *The Downtown Review* 5, no. 2 (2019): https://engagedscholarship.csuohio.edu/tdr/vol5/iss2/4.

△

There are three parts to an emergency room visit: triage, treatment, and disposition.

Triage is a brief assessment, usually by a nurse, to categorize your ailment as emergent, urgent, or nonurgent. Nonurgent means you're stable and at low risk for becoming unstable. Nonurgent patients may have a long wait, during which they can become unstable.

During the treatment phase you see the doctor or mid-level provider (a nurse practitioner or physician's assistant). They order tests, medicine, and maybe breathing treatments, and then you wait.

Disposition is made when your treatment is concluded. Based on the results and reassessment, you're discharged home, admitted to the hospital, or transferred to another care facility.

ERs study this flow of activity to identify the "time sucks" and reduce inefficiencies. When ERs are inefficient, it's not just resources and services being jeopardized, but the health and lives of patients. Eventually I joined the ER management team and got to be part of the hunt for solutions to improve ER flow.

Before electronic charting, data collection was clunky, often achieved by tedious manual chart reviews. We charted by paper when I started in the ER. When I left twenty-nine years later, we were on our third computer charting system for tracking patients and documenting medical interventions.

Electronic systems greatly enhanced our ability to identify patterns of behavior that created bottlenecks. The only thing more important than flow of patient care is the quality of the care, and if you don't have decent flow, then you risk delaying that care. The best care delivered too late is worth nothing—hence flow and quality are intertwined.

The patient most at risk is the one waiting, the one not fully assessed, who may have something going on that ER staff doesn't suspect—and what the ER doesn't know about you could kill you.

However, if it's not likely to kill you today or this week, then they're going to limit how hard they look. This is why you may not get a CT scan or MRI even if you ultimately need it to diagnose or rule out a condition. You will only get it as part of your ER visit if the information is needed emergently. That's because they have limited rooms and staff, and the longer they take to assess potentially harmful conditions, the longer it takes to get to that next waiting patient, and that waiting patient may have a condition trying to kill them today.

△

Social workers, too, can think of their work in terms of three: preparation, interaction, and closure. Even in the ER, where interventions are about as short-term as they come, you prepare by reviewing a chart and perhaps gathering resource information, then you meet the patient and family to explore their situation and discuss what you can offer. You go away to do what you said you'd do and then conclude your interaction by making your last visit before they leave or get admitted. You go to the doctor and nurse to summarize what you did for their patient and always document it in the chart.

Among the essential aspects of social work practice taught in school, I found these three to be the most relevant in the ER: unconditional positive regard, patient autonomy, and detachment.

Unconditional positive regard means that I maintain a level of respect for patients, independent of their character and beliefs, and that I want the best for them regardless of who and how they are. Unconditional positive regard is a concept you embody, not declare. My coworkers would have rolled their eyes if I defended the patient who verbally abused us. If I tried to explain how a patient's desperation could be the fuel of their anger, how we, the ER staff, can look like every other person that failed this patient, my coworkers would have felt betrayed by me, and I'd lose their trust. We do not have to be doormats or allow abusive behavior; we can hold patients accountable. We can set limits, clarify boundaries, communicate what we won't tolerate, and still want the patient to get better, and want to take reasonable steps to help them. Not taking the patient's behavior personally is the key.

Ms. Mitchum was an elderly woman who came in periodically for breathing treatments. She lived alone and needed help at home and transportation to medical appointments, but every time anyone came in her room who wasn't dressed in scrubs, she shouted, "Are you a social worker? I don't want a social worker!" If you answered in the affirmative, she unleashed her fury, screaming until you left the room. She wouldn't tell any of us (even those wearing scrubs) what she had against social workers, but obviously she did not trust them. Her mistrust was an obstacle, but not a reason to give up. We did whatever we could for her behind the scenes, including arranging a way home.

No one expects the patient to be in a good mood—we realize they are in pain and afraid. Being in the ER is the worst-case scenario for the patient and family; hence, we tend to see their worst behavior. Some patients or family members who lost their tempers would later apologize, as they saw we continued to do everything we could for them. I told them that we know the ER is a stressful place, a place they did not expect or want to be. We know they are not at their best. Being at our best, despite the patient's behavior, is what we expect of ourselves. Believing in unconditional positive regard is easy. Embodying it constantly is impossible.

Once I was called to a room to talk to a patient about a bus pass. I found Ms. Butler in a wheelchair. She was thin, with a red face—maybe rosacea, maybe just from anger or stress. She had on jeans that were big for her small frame and a T-shirt from a taco chain. She looked like she was in her fifties, but she could've been closer to thirty. I recognized her. Some days she parked her wheelchair in a triangle of concrete in the middle of a busy street during rush hour, holding up a sign I never read as I drove past.

Bus passes cost the hospital money. We don't want a patient to assume they can have one every time they come to the ER, so we ask them about their situation. We document the information and our actions in the chart, so an advocate will see it the next time the patient comes in and determine if we should provide another.

Ms. Butler told me she was sent to the ER because her blood sugar was high. She had access to free insulin—brownie points to whoever helped her jump through those hoops—but now that she had exceeded the maximum time she could stay in the shelter, she was in the woods, with no place to keep the insulin chilled.

She was frustrated, no, actually she was raging, totally pissed off that she was in this wheelchair as a result of having her feet "cut on" by a doctor who thought the "easiest" solution was to cut the entire foot off. She's down half of one foot and two digits on the other—so far. And that bus pass? I was going to give it to her, but first I said, "We can't do this every time."

She cut me off, telling me I could just keep it. "If I can't get to and from the wound care clinic regularly, then I just have to have my damn feet cut off or have nothing done and die."

I begged her to accept the pass and gave her my contact information so we could make a long-range plan.

She'd been turned down for disability. She knew this was insane. "It's the kind of thing that makes people walk into theaters and shoot people; they just snap." She wouldn't let me give her another source to help with the disability; she already owed money to an attorney, who told her she couldn't switch to anyone else.

She took the bus pass. I stepped out to tell the nurse she was ready for discharge. A young woman, the patient's visitor, walked in and started yelling at the patient, then ran out. The patient raged that the young woman ran off with her ID and food stamps, and wheeled herself out in pursuit, not staying for discharge papers.

The next day I drove past her in that triangle of concrete. Still, I didn't read her sign, and I didn't look her in the eyes.

Extensive efforts were made by other hospital departments to help this patient with her steadily worsening diabetes and lack of housing. Missing appointments at the diabetes clinic caused her to bounce back into the ER, where getting her insulin became our problem. Her substance abuse and explosive temperament made her hard to work with, one of the most troublesome patients that year, but eventually she got into community clinics and housing, thanks to many helping professionals working together patiently for countless hours.

I don't expect a diabetic, disabled, and unhoused person to be cheerful. You could spend all day trying to parse out how much of her situation she was accountable for. But that wouldn't change the current situation and just wastes time. If you manage to rationalize to yourself why you should do less for her, you put her in more jeopardy and increase the chance of her returning in even worse shape. My regret is that in our first meeting, after hearing just part of her story, I went into default mode—handing her the pass with the accompanying lecture—instead of asking to hear the whole story.

Patient autonomy is a social work tenet that would garner support from ER coworkers—at least theoretically. We all say that we uphold a client's or patient's right to make their own choices, but often when a patient exercises that right, we condemn them—both when they decline treatment and when they choose to pursue treatment that appears futile.

Changing a person's mind about a health decision is possible but takes time, and the clock is always ticking in the ER. Patient and family need time to receive information and process it. Still, we give it a shot. A doctor pairs up with a social worker to try to convince a patient to stay or be admitted, or to explain why admission isn't necessary.

When a patient tries to be agreeable yet doesn't want to comply with our recommendation, they counter with a "Yes, but." They have a reason why your plan will not work for them. Come up with a solution to that problem and you'll hear another "Yes, but."

When social workers hear this phrase, we should know to back up, to start over from the patient's definition of the problem and look for a patient-defined solution. But in the ER, there's no time to quibble about options. From medical staff's perspective, they understand the problem and have the answers; it's the patient's job to accept the solution. So, when a referral is made that doesn't work for the patient, or they can't pay for the treatment, or they don't have transportation, that's not medicine's problem. That's where social workers step in.

A third tenet of social work, detachment, helped me survive these grim realities. It's a coping mechanism and a technique.

A social work professor used to say, "Don't let your helping get in the way of your *helping.*" One of my classmates in the undergraduate program of social work dropped out after a few semesters for this very reason. She said she couldn't do the work; she felt it too deeply. It may seem absurd, but caring can get in the way of caregiving.

When she left the program, I was floored. Dropping out never occurred to me. I realized that some aspects of social work might be too hard for me. My solution was to strike off categories like child protective services and foster care, because if you made a mistake in those jobs, a child suffered. I assumed I could work around any other areas of significant discomfort.

Growing up in a military family, I knew not to get too attached to people, places, and even pets, because we moved so frequently. Like most helping professionals, I see my childhood as early training.

There is an unspoken expectation on the military family unit to meet all the needs of the individual members. Kids don't have the continuity of a community they've grown up in, friends and neighbors they've known for years. Parents can't lean on longtime friends to hear their frustrations and worries, to advise or comfort them. Extended family is usually only seen once or twice a year, less if you're stationed overseas.

With unfamiliar local resources and few social networks not related to the military, there's a weighted dependency of family members on the family unit. Military families extract what they need from each other. My earliest memories involve a panicky feeling of being unmoored, at risk of floating away. I felt the most anchored when I was physically close to home but with a degree of emotional separation.

As a college social work intern at a psychiatric facility, I joined a weeklong education program for family members of patients in the addiction unit. One handout we received was titled *Detachment.*

It described a way to live with an addict and avoid much of the usual conflict. You learn to identify what is and what is not within your control. You cannot stop your loved one from using, from lying, from suffering, but you can choose your own actions. It is a way to manage your expectations, frustration, and angst. A way to accept the person you loved irrespective of their addiction. You can love them, but you cannot change them. You are not responsible for their actions. I could apply it immediately. I still lived with my first husband, who was an alcoholic, and of course I didn't want him to be.

Detachment came easily to me because it built on a foundation I'd created as a child. I'd spent my childhood yearning to be an adult, to have some agency over my life. And now here I was, a college student with a coveted adult professional skill already tucked in my back pocket.

I believed I had this detachment thing down. It helped with my family, it helped me survive that failed marriage, and in the ER, detachment helped me deflect the intense emotions of patients and families. I could sympathize with their pain and fear without absorbing it.

Years later, the books I read on meditation philosophy encouraged the cultivation of detachment, and I greeted it like an old friend, never confessing my fear that my degree of fluency kept me from deep connection.

$$\triangle$$

Developmental psychologist Erik Erikson divided the human lifespan into eight stages of healthy development, proposing a major challenge at each stage.[3]

In order, they are: Trust vs. Mistrust, Autonomy vs. Shame and Doubt, Initiative vs. Guilt, Industry vs. Inferiority, Identity vs. Role Confusion, Intimacy vs. Isolation, Generativity vs. Stagnation, and Integrity vs. Despair.

I encountered his theory as an undergraduate. I liked the packaging of these stages. They seemed orderly and precise. They let me know the task at hand and the consequence of failure. They suggested a reason for dysfunction and frustration—a challenge left uncompleted or done completely wrong.

The last time I applied them to my life I was in my twenties, when I was nowhere close to the last stages. I snuck a peek at those later

---

3. Erik Erikson, *Identity and the Life Cycle* (W. W. Norton & Company, 1994).

challenges, but it was like jumping to the end of a book—I lacked the context, the experience of the journey. Those last three stages—Intimacy vs. Isolation, Generativity vs. Stagnation, and Integrity vs. Despair—span middle age to old age.

I return to them now the way I rewatch a classic movie—to compare its personal impact and meaning through the lens of years passed. Now, when I rewatch the activist woman in *The Way We Were* leave the conventional (but gorgeous) man, my older self cheers her resolve, whereas my preteen self mourned the loss of their romance.

Almost forty years had passed since I applied Erikson's stages to myself. I wanted to see how I measured up to the challenges of middle and older adulthood.

I had a happy marriage of over thirty-five years, so check off Intimacy? I had a productive career and produced two children; is that Generativity in the bag? Integrity—making meaning of it all—that was the real stumper. Is there a secret formula to find meaning and stave off despair, and is that formula available to an ordinary human?

I could have shrugged off Erikson, but instead, I did what we all do these days—I googled him. I went looking for modern voices that reached back to his work from the 1950s to bring his wisdom forward into our lives today. Were his stages still relevant to the modern world? Were his stages relevant to me?

Google led me to Dr. Ruthellen Josselson, whose books on women's identity spring from her own examination of Erikson. She discovered that his case studies and biographies regard men exclusively, so she embarked on her own meaning making.

Josselson followed a group of women for thirty-five years, looking at what shaped their identities, the central challenge of Erikson's fifth stage. She interviewed these women at ages twenty-one, thirty-three, forty-three, and fifty-five, beginning in 1972. And, in terms of identity, Josselson finds that gender matters. She also notes that while youth and old age have been well examined, we know less about the middle years of life.[4]

---

4. Ruthellen Josselson, *Paths to Fulfillment* (Oxford University Press, 2017).

Josselson writes that for these women "identity is expressed in the quality of connection with those one loves."[5] She acknowledges she is confirming work that has preceded hers: "Nearly all researchers who have intensely studied women conclude that interconnection is the foundation of identity . . . yet psychology persists in thinking about identity in individualistic terms."[6]

This interplay between identity and connection is reinforced in social work teaching. The client or patient is considered in regard to their environment, as part of a web of family, culture, and values. To separate them from this ecology is to deny the bigger picture of what influences their beliefs and behavior, what makes them unique.

Patients, female and male, rarely make health care decisions based on what is best for them alone, yet the ER wants to keep things simple and focus solely on the individual and the medical problem at hand. Josselson states that "our experience of identity rests on a sense of fit between self and the social world, on the expectation that the environment will, at least much of the time, be in tune with us." Here was a new insight: The way the ER worked, and the version of reality it unveiled, was not in tune with my professional or personal life. Everything I valued about how to work with people, my sense of security and belief in a benevolent universe, got upended. There was a limit to how much I could change the ER, so I went to work on myself.

△

As I recall my time in the ER, I see myself moving through three phases, leaning heavily on a particular attribute in each phase. These attributes define the phases of my journey: Imagine, Act, Listen.

Using Joseph Campbell's hero structure, Imagine is my call to the journey, Act is the journey itself, and Listen is my return home.

I don't recommend this route—it's rather catawampus. But it's the way I coped, how I traveled through middle adulthood, age

5. Josselson, *Paths to Fulfillment*, 274.
6. Josselson, *Paths to Fulfillment*, 289. She cites: "Franz & Stewart, 1994, Gilligan, 1982; Miller, 1976, Chodorow, 1978; Hulbert and Schuster, 1993, among others."

twenty-eight to fifty-seven—my tenure in the ER. One story evokes another, related more by theme than by a timeline. My categories are not tidy; they leak out at the edges. This is what happens when you try to wedge a human life into a structure. I feel myself going in circles—I hope it's a spiral and that as I go around, I'm learning, climbing higher. But because I am part of the structure, I cannot see my path clearly.

As Dante famously begins *The Divine Comedy*, "In the middle of the road of life, I found myself in a dark forest, where the straight path was confusing." In my fifties, my "middle road of life," I went seeking the path out of that forest, to see where I was and how I got there, so that I could move forward. I wrote this book.

Dante went to a great deal more trouble than I'm willing to take on. What I've described here is not nine circles of hell, but it is the experience of nearly twenty-nine years in one ER.

IMAGINE

In the Crazy

The ER is a place tucked far away from the minds of people in the regular world—except, perhaps, when choosing underwear.

If mothers still issue warnings about underwear—the lack or the sorry state of it, as a risk to good reputation—then perhaps you've thought about the ER when you reach toward the back of the drawer. If you have a medical emergency and end up in the ER, those undies will be pulled down by a stranger and tossed on the floor for all to see.

I didn't upgrade my undie drawer until the ER became my employer. The ER was no longer full of strangers. I couldn't bear thoughts of my coworkers' smirks and snickering asides if they saw my white granny panties.

Patients are in the ER because their worst-case scenario is playing out. They've had an accident, gotten suddenly sick, or their chronic illness is worse at a time when their doctor or therapist cannot see them—like a Friday afternoon, a weekend, an evening, or a holiday. Or, if they have no doctor and/or no insurance, they end up in the ER due to a lack of alternatives, which is also a worst-case scenario.

The ER is also where you go when someone you love is missing. You think, *Worst-case scenario, they're at the hospital.* And when you're ready to call the hospital, you start with the ER.

But there are worse places your loved one could be. If they're in the ER at least they are found, even if we don't yet know who they are or how to reach you. They're being cared for, even if we don't know their medical history or exactly what to do for them yet.

Worse would be your loved one hurt and alone, or dead in a place no one knows to look; or they could stay missing—probably because they left you. It sounds harsh and extreme, but I know these are real possibilities because they are the real experiences of ER patients and families.

△

My role as patient advocate in the emergency room of a regional hospital started as a part-time job. It didn't require my master's degree and didn't pay as much as my job in adoptions, but it was steady work with benefits. I kept my adoption job and added ER shifts on the weekends, when my husband could stay with the kids.

The position was newish to the hospital, having been created by an innovative ER director and then expanded by the next director, the one who hired me. Both were seeking to soften the impact of the experience of an ER visit on patients and their families. My director wanted the advocates to do more. She wanted the ER to be less dependent on hospital departments outside of the ER.

The needs of an ER patient are immediate and acute *even when they aren't*, because a patient in an ER room is taking up space that another patient needs. ERs must often depend on other departments for services: Phlebotomy for labs, Radiology for X-rays, Transport for moving patients upstairs. When I started, we also depended on other departments for reporting child abuse, resolving complex social service issues, and providing postmortem services.

Stat is a medical term from the Latin word *statim*, meaning immediately. Everything is stat in the ER. When we called these other departments or put in an order, they sometimes had the audacity to hold our request in the order they received it. This reflects a basic misunderstanding of how the ER works. When we called them to explain what *stat* meant, we were told, "The ER thinks they're special." But waiting for our turn meant our patients waited, keeping our treatment rooms full, impairing our ability to care for the next heart attack or trauma. Our waiting rooms filled—delaying the delivery of care to patients who might have been unstable.

Delays can lead to patients leaving without being seen (LWOBS). An LWOBS patient has only received a brief triage assessment. They need a full medical assessment to know if they have a serious condition. Patients who stay long enough to come back to a room for a medical exam but leave without completing treatment (LWOCT) are also at risk.

I was always impressed that hospital administrators knew our LWOBS and LWOCT rates, believing it indicated their commitment and concern for our patients. But a few years in, my ER director pointed out the less rosy motivation—it's also a loss in potential revenue. The hospital bears the cost of staff, equipment, and the building. To survive, it has to be able to bill for services, and they can't bill for services not received. My position existed not only because it was good for patients and families but because it was a potential revenue enhancer—providing a better ER experience might positively influence their hospital choice in the future.

When a patient dies, risk to other patients can increase, because a death in the department usually adds a delay to care for the living. No one likes to think of it in this way, but for the sake of patient safety, it is a reality we cannot ignore.

Our ER lessened this risk of delay by minimizing the nonmedical postmortem tasks required of doctors and nurses. Those services include offering comfort and assistance to the families; ensuring that the coroner, organ procurement entity, and funeral home are notified promptly, with documentation completed; and setting up transport to the morgue.

When I started, advocates covered the ER for only twelve hours a day. But patients don't die in cooperation with a schedule. Eventually the ER advocates were scheduled twenty hours a day, and we were called in as needed between three and seven a.m. As a result, the ER became independent of other social service departments. We trained each other about community resources for patients and how to make reports of elder and child abuse or neglect. We learned when we were required to contact the police and how to get a patient a sexual assault exam from the county forensic team. The advocate role improved patient services and prevented delays. We became a respected part of the ER team.

△

Anyone can come to the ER for anything, but I don't recommend it. For those who can't afford to see a primary care doctor regularly, the ER may be where you go to get medication for your allergies, get some advice about that low back pain, have that hangnail removed—all frequent presenting complaints of patients seen daily.

Presents is one of many words with multiple applications in the medical profession. How a patient presents can refer to the way they arrived (*"presents by private vehicle/ambulance/police"*), or to who came with them (*"presents with her husband"*), or to their condition (*"presents with hypertension, confusion, unresponsive"*). Once they present at our threshold, no matter the manner or condition, we are obligated to care for them. Ideally this creates a level playing field whereby anyone can present; have a triage screening of their vitals, history, and immediate issue; be placed in the appropriate category; and then be seen in the order dictated by that category.

It's not a first-come, first-served situation. If you are stable, you may lose your place in line because there is no definitive line. The queue is fluid. The sickest are seen first, and if you get sicker as you wait, you should move up in priority.

ER staff is not without biases and prejudices, and despite training and education to increase self-awareness and insight, ER social workers are no exception. Patients could be minimized or discounted due to who they were or what they looked like, but at that time I believed a patient's numbers were an equalizer that penetrated biases, because that's what I most commonly saw.

Those numbers are your vital signs: your temperature, heart rate, respiratory rate, and blood pressure, compared to another number: your age. Along with more nuanced observations—level of orientation, breath sounds, your stated level of pain—these numbers dictate the next step of care.

Along with emergent, urgent, and nonurgent categories of patient ailments, there are public health diseases of varying severity that present to the limited resources of the ER.

When I came to the ER in the early nineties, I assumed treating patients with AIDS would be a huge concern for the staff. But universal precautions had been introduced in the late eighties. The staff was confident they could provide care and stay safe as long as they followed protocols. My coworkers were much more concerned about contracting tuberculosis, which is transmitted by air. We didn't have negative-pressure rooms in our ER for TB patients until a few years after I arrived.

The next big public health disease, MRSA (Methicillin-resistant Staphylococcus aureus), wasn't widespread in our community until the early 2000s. Although usually mild and treatable in healthy people, MRSA is also devilishly easy to transmit and can lead to a serious, life-threatening infection, as it is resistant to antibiotic treatment. Some ER staff contracted MRSA, and most cases resolved easily. I was told that working in the ER meant that most of us probably carried it, but unless we had an active breakout, we were not infectious.

Universal precautions became standard precautions. When training new nonmedical staff, my spiel about staying safe at work included information about these transmittable diseases, as well as nonviolent conflict resolution. Like me, they were surprised at what the ER revealed about this North Georgia community: We have a large unhoused population. We have victims of stabbings and gunshot wounds. The mental health needs of our community vastly exceed the resources. We have public health diseases barely contained. There are frequent cases of child and elder abuse, domestic violence, and rape. Though we see the worst of a community, we know this is just a sampler, the cases that came to our door. Working in the ER exposes staff to violence and risk of infection, in addition to exhaustion and despair.

△

Getting hired for the ER in any role means that someone believes you have what it takes to work in a fast-paced, unpredictable environment. You have to be prepared to do your job and more—with that "more" being undefined and infinite.

When a secretary is the only one who sees the suicidal patient slip out the back door, she grabs her phone and follows him, calling others as she keeps an eye on where he goes. A supply tech is enlisted to hold a combative patient so an IV line can be started. A social worker and security staff place a patient's body in a bag because the nurses are too busy and there's a patient waiting for that room.

There is always a patient waiting, even when there is not. You can be surprised by nothing only if you are ready for anything. This is the essential mindset.

Ancillary staff, registrars, transporters, and lab and X-ray technicians are sometimes assigned to the ER as punishment. If someone doesn't like you, they know the ER will either make you or break you— it may drive you out of the hospital altogether. But sometimes a person rises to the challenge and stays. They find their people in the ER, their place in the crazy.

The staff in ERs share a commitment to see whoever presents. In one hour, doctors and nurses can go from treating a sore throat to intubating a patient whose throat is closing. Given the choice, they prefer the intubation. They want to provide emergency care, not primary care. But primary care was part of the gig for as long as I worked there.

Staff members try to manage their frustration, to not take it out on the patients, and mostly they succeed. I know this because when they failed, I was the one who heard about it and was expected to soothe the offended patient.

Yet despite these challenges, the ER is a destination of choice for medical staff. It's not where a doctor lands late in their career, or where a nurse goes after years of office practice. It is the place where they start if they're lucky enough to get in. They tend to be young and energetic, and if they're going to stay, they have to stay smart, adaptive, and hardworking.

If you find yourself belted on to a hard backboard from the scene of a car accident, remember that this is not actually the worst-case scenario. You could be in the morgue or lying hidden and unconscious in a ditch. Your accident was unlucky, but where you landed was fortunate: the faces that hover over you are the faces of people who want to be there—they got in, they made the cut, and they are working hard to stay. This may be one of the worst days of your life, but they're in their element.

They are the ones who adapted to working in a place that fundamentally shifts one's perception of reality, where a normal day is full of patients having crises. What couldn't, shouldn't, wouldn't ever happen *does* happen—and it's just a Tuesday. This upending of normalcy drives some staff away. The short-timers are so numerous that their existence is just a blip in our memory. They couldn't handle the chaos, the emotions, the range of skills needed. They couldn't handle the impossible shifts, the unrelenting busyness, or just didn't "get" us, our way of doing things, seeing things, our humor. We hurt their feelings, and they didn't get over it.

That file of short-timers gets thick quickly, and if their memory is invoked at all, it is only as a reminder of how special we are, the ER careerists. Those that don't leave in their first month, week, or even after their first shift are those that find something addictive in the crazy, in the way that they fit into it.

Of those long-timers, there are two groups. The first group sees through the ER's strange appeal. They recognize that staying too long exacts too big a sacrifice. They stay a few years, to prove to themselves they can do it and earn some solid skills.

Laura, one of my closest nurse friends, cut back on her shifts so she could take classes. Once she became a nurse practitioner, she quit the ER to join a cardiologist's practice. She no longer worked nights, holidays, or weekends. She got better working conditions and consistently garnered the respect that she always deserved.

She was one of the smart ones, getting out before it was too late, in time to have a different life, to be a different person. I was not one of the smart ones.

I didn't envy her or the advocates who left to become counselors or work in hospice or county services. Maybe it's part of that flawed perception of mine, but I suspected then, and still do, that they missed the ER, that it was a high point in their life, that they envied us, the second group, those who stayed behind.

Hidden Drive

I'd forgotten how long Laurel Lane was. Just outside the city limits, bisecting two highways, it's lined with modest seventies-era ranches and split-levels. I had been working in the ER for about five years when an eight-year-old boy rolled down one of these driveways on his bike and out into the street, where he was struck by a car. I used to live close to his street, but only drove it one previous time, a few days after he came in.

Anthony was my first pediatric death. He was younger than my children but went to the same school. The principal knew me and that I worked in the ER. I don't remember if she knew I was part of his care team. She asked me to speak to the parents at a PTA meeting a few days later. I spoke about grief in children, because all their children, whether or not they knew Anthony, knew they'd lost a schoolmate. I don't recall what I said, but I do remember feeling that it was inadequate.

I went to his funeral. The church was packed with mourners wearing their grief raw, unmasked. The church swayed with music and wails and tears. Older ladies whirled around the family and congregation, watching for those needing help, those overcome with emotion. They knew their role—they had done this many times before. It was my first time attending a funeral in a church of Black congregants, but not my last. Anthony's parents were there, of course, but that's not where my memory holds them.

△

As Anthony arrived by ambulance and the staff did CPR, I met his parents in the lobby and took them to the Family Room. The father insisted I take him to his son. In those days I had to ask permission to bring back any visitor to a trauma patient. I asked the doctor. He told me to keep them out.

As I went to deliver this message of "No, not yet," the father strode right past me to find his son's room on his own. I was relieved. Keeping families out sickened me. I knew what I'd want in his place, what I'd demand. If your child is fighting for their life, there is nothing more important than being by their side. But in an ER, everything is subordinated to medical care unless or until the patient dies or recovers. If the doctor believes that family at the bedside could interfere with that care, then the family can't be at the bedside—they call this "putting the patient first."

The room was easy to find. It was a big trauma room in the middle of the ER, and the walls were glass. The father rushed in. There were about ten people in the room: nurses pushing medicines, nurses and medics working together to find more veins to push more medicines, techs hooking the patient up to monitors, X-ray techs and the blood bank standing by, and the doctor at the bedside watching the monitor as CPR continued. But no matter how consumed they were with their task, they all felt it when the father entered the room. His silent terror was a wave that simultaneously crashed into all of them. I stumbled in behind him and watched as the doctor, nurses, and techs turned tensely to look first at him, then at me, to see how this was going to go.

△

Staff doesn't expect any parent to be able to watch what they do to children. Early in my career, a doctor shut me down when I advocated for parents to be in the room as we pumped the stomach of their daughter who'd eaten adult medication. That doctor said that every parent wants to be with their child at such a time, but "No one can watch that happen to their child, I don't care who you are." He felt it was our job to set those boundaries for the parents. I kept my mouth shut, though I knew from experience he was wrong.

My daughter was two when she was hospitalized with pneumonia. I wasn't working in the ER yet. I made the two-hour drive to Atlanta that day for my job in adoptions, to file paperwork to ensure a baby's medical costs would be covered, thereby enhancing his chance of being adopted. I'd only just been alerted that the deadline was that day, the same day my daughter woke up seeming a little puny.

I wanted to stay home with my daughter, but no one else could file that paperwork. If that paperwork didn't go in, his adoption would almost certainly be delayed. Having to search for parents who could pay the expenses would make the difference between him going quickly to a forever home or spending months in foster care—his welfare up against my daughter's. But my daughter had a father, and this infant in foster care had only me—I couldn't *not* go.

Most of my work in adoptions was making home study and post-placement visits with families, a task that could easily be rescheduled. But this documentation task fell to me because I had worked with the birth mom throughout her pregnancy—something I rarely did and never did again, due to my discomfort. I worried about my (unintended) influence on the mom to keep or relinquish her child, and if she relinquished, the subsequent stress around getting her child placed in a family was too intense.

I came home from Atlanta to find my friend with our three-year-old son. Our daughter had gotten worse. My husband had taken her to the pediatrician, who had admitted her to the hospital. The friend kept our son as I tore down the road to the hospital, and raced to her room on the pediatric floor. She had an IV in her arm. My husband gave me a gentle but resolute look. He stepped away to update me and calmly relayed the horror of getting an IV into her as she screamed.

"The nurse wasn't able to get an IV, so she came back with another nurse and a board. They said I would have to step out as they strapped her on the board to get her IV started. I told them that was fine, but I was staying. They didn't like it, but they let me stay. I held her other hand. They strapped her on to the board so she couldn't move. She looked at me and jerked her head toward the door, pleading, 'Daddy, out! Daddy, out!' She wanted me to pick her up and run through the door . . . It was terrible. But now they know. If that IV comes out, they'll do that again, but we've established that we're staying in the room. You have to stay in the room."

He wanted me to steel myself in case this happened on my watch. We'd have to take turns being in the hospital and being at home with our son. I was still squeamish, but that no longer mattered. My husband had set a precedent with the nurses: Yes, we were *those* kinds of parents, the ones who would stay with her no matter what. He'd drawn that line, and we would hold it.

When the IV line fell out of her arm and they had to start another, we were both there. It was undisputedly my turn. It wasn't fair to ask him to stand in for me. But he did, taking on that trauma a second time rather than inflicting it on me.

Weeks later he told me: "I thought being there while they started that IV would make her hate me, that she would associate me with being held down and stuck, for not picking her up and taking her away, but I think it's made us closer. She knows that I was there, I stayed by her side."

Up until then she'd been a mommy's girl. This part of this story, the part where she gets closer to her dad, and maybe a tiny bit less close to me—this part doesn't bother me at all. I knew it was in everyone's best interest for us to be interchangeable, for both children to be equally secure and content with either of us. We shuddered often at the idea of shouldering parenting alone, a seeming impossibility that is the daily reality of single parents.

△

Anthony lay unresponsive on the gurney with staff clustered around him. His tall father dropped to his knees, an action so primal and honest that I wanted to join him there, but I was aware of the staff's unease—and part of my job was to keep the staff comfortable, which meant making them believe I had some control of the situation, though clearly, I had none.

I approached, but he flung his arms out. "Don't touch me! Leave me alone." As he knelt in the middle of the room, I brought his wife in, Anthony's mother. Not only did I want her there for Anthony, but I thought maybe she could reach the dad and get him off the floor.

It seems absurd that his kneeling on the floor mattered at all, but there are several reasons we don't want someone on the floor in the ER. One, the floor is dirty, no matter how recently it was cleaned. Two, a person on the floor is in the way—machines have to roll in, and the gurney may have to roll out, and staff is rushing around and could trip over them. Three, if you're on the floor in the ER, something is wrong with you, and you're surrounded by a team of fixers. Also, four, once you're on the floor, it's harder to control you, to take you by the arm and drag you off or push you down into a wheelchair and roll you away.

When the wife came in, she took in the scene, her child barely visible through the cluster of staff around the bed. She went to her husband, but again his arms went out. "Don't touch me." She stood in the back of the room, crying. I stood beside her, my hand lightly on her arm. The doctor went from one parent to the other, crouching down to talk to the dad, to explain what had been done and the futility of continuing.

When I remember Anthony, I remember this: his parents, the people who loved him the most, starkly separate, each in a place so hellish the other could not reach them.

When our daughter got sick as a teenager from an ailment that defied quick diagnosis, before we knew what it was and the extent of the damage, the anxiety and anguish divided my husband and me. Our fears were so thick we couldn't find one another.

All the bad things that happen to families, to children—accidents, new diagnoses of terrible diseases—in my world, these things happened all the time. What if it was just our turn? The image of Anthony's parents, years ago, in that room, broken by grief, came to me over and over. Did we fight together to stay at her side when she was young only to stand apart now and cry alone? The two people who shared the deepest love for her, now unable to give each other basic comfort?

Soon after Anthony's death, I drove down Laurel Lane. I wanted to see where he had lived, to understand how he could be fatally hit on a street I had thought was straight and flat and clear.

It starts that way, from the four-lane highway—tidy lawns for unassuming houses. But soon it begins to ramble, dipping up and down around curves as the trees get bigger. Only the sign, "Hidden Drive," hints at what you needed to know sooner. I don't know if Anthony's parents still live here, or even if they still live together at all.

Laurel Lane ends at a country highway, where there now stands a roadside memorial. Someone else died on this road. I don't know their story, and the people who placed that cross and flowers probably do not know Anthony's, but knowing that others may travel this road in sad remembrance makes the drive less lonely. As if I belong to a fellowship of travelers, making sad, secret pilgrimages separately, but linked in knowing this road hides tragedy.

A Good Trauma

People get hurt every day. When ER nurses say they want "a good trauma," they are not wishing others bad luck; they simply want one of those bad things to coincide with their shift. A fan of car racing wouldn't say they want someone to get hurt, but if a crash is going to happen, they'd like it to happen when they can see it.

In the ER, a patient that rolls in with a complex and emergent condition tests staff's skills and knowledge against the pressure of a ticking clock. New equipment may get unveiled, or a procedure performed that they've only heard about. The frenzied action requires such concentration that it's only after the patient is rolled out of the room that they look at each other, in a post-endorphin daze, dimly aware that time has passed but with no idea how much. Then they look around at what they've done to their surroundings.

The room tells the story—the messier it is, the more satisfied they seem. The floor takes the brunt of the abuse: Packaging from sterile equipment lies where it was thrown, along with countless bits of peelings from adhesive stickers, patches, perhaps a syringe or two, tubing, and blood. The blood is in drops, spatters, swirls, and puddles. Anything that got in the way was flung down: a sheet, clothing, shoes. A nurse or tech winds their way around the room, picking up the detritus of lifesaving efforts, mumbling apologies to environmental services as they come in with a mop.

Staff's eagerness for a good trauma serves the patients. Those who enjoy working traumas are usually the best at it. They seek the chance to practice and are rewarded with the ultimate rush of making a difference, saving a life. But even when a trauma has a bad outcome for the patient, the experience is helpful, instructive, yielding lessons that benefit the next patient.

A trauma is a spinning vortex. Navigating inside gives you a sense of mastery and power. Everyone's job is more clearly delineated than usual, which creates a sense of rhythm. You fall into the flow state of extreme focus and timelessness. Even advocates sometimes desire the occasional trauma as a break from the monotony of rounding rooms, explaining delays, and coordinating transport home.

Mr. Sims came in on a Saturday, found by a neighbor. While cleaning out gutters on a summer morning, he slipped off the ladder and fell onto his concrete driveway. His wife was running errands, both of them getting their chores done before the Georgia heat took off. But Mr. Sims wasn't found until the afternoon. His neighbor saw the ladder on its side before he saw Mr. Sims splayed in the driveway, surrounded by blood from his head wound.

The neighbor tried to rouse him but wisely did not try to move him. Mr. Sims was unconscious and remained unconscious, so we never really met. I followed the stretcher into the room to hear the paramedics' report. Strapped on to a backboard with a cervical collar to stabilize his neck, his gray hair rusted with blood. The tech removed what remained of his T-shirt, cut apart by the medics. Tattered, blood-streaked strips were wadded into a ball and handed to me. Not wearing gloves, I used the plastic patient belongings bag to catch the shirt. Trauma shears cut off the pants to minimize tugging or moving any body parts that may have been injured. As I collected the clothing from the tech, everyone in the room listened to the report, which included mechanism and timing of injury, injuries known and suspected, vital signs, and medical interventions on the scene and in the truck as they sped to the hospital.

The report included mention of the neighbor. Once the doctor finished asking his questions, the medics caught my silent inquiry, adding: "Patient's married, and the neighbor will inform his wife when she gets home."

I left the bag of clothes in a corner of the room and went to the lobby, where a visitor assistant was stationed behind the locked doors leading to ER treatment rooms. When the front knows what's happening in the back, they are better able to respond to the wide-eyed loved one rushing in. Even a little bit of information can help them calm the frantic family member: *"Yes, Mr. Sims is here. The doctor is assessing him, and I'll let them know you're here, and we'll get you back there as soon as we can."*

To hear immediately that they are in the right place and their loved one is being cared for takes their anxiety down a tiny notch. Keeping the front staff informed also helps them brace for that wave of emotional intensity coming their way. They have to stay focused to gather information—how the visitor is related to the patient, whether they are intact enough to come to the back. The visitor assistant has to mentally psych themselves up for delaying an impassioned plea to see their loved one—which will come immediately and almost always be denied.

After I spoke with the visitor assistant, I returned to my duties for other patients. It's easy to get sucked into a trauma, to stay in the room to witness the excited flurry of activity, but when family isn't yet there but is supposedly on their way, we have a few minutes to help other patients waiting for discharge. Once the family of a trauma patient is in the ER, we may not be available for an hour or more, so toggling between tasks, helping to empty rooms so we can bring more patients back from the lobby, is essential to facilitate the flow of patients.

I took note of the time. If the wife didn't arrive in a few minutes, then I'd need to play detective to ensure she got the message and was coming. When someone calls 911, the ambulance service has the number of the phone, so that would be the place to start, but as I was in a room explaining follow-up resources to a patient, I got the call from the lobby. I finished quickly and rushed to the patient's room to get an update. The room was empty; the patient was getting a CT scan and X-rays. I found the primary nurse and confirmed that Mr. Sims was still unconscious but stable. I hurried to the lobby, where the wife stood so close to the locked automated door that it almost hit her as I came out. The visitor assistant at the desk nodded—this was Mrs. Sims.

I introduced myself and confirmed her identity. I told her I was going to take her back—it was important to say that right away because that's what she was listening for, and she wouldn't hear anything else until I said it. "I'm going to take you back to his room, but right now he's in a CT scan, where they're checking for injuries. He'll be back in a few minutes. He's not conscious, but his vital signs are stable. He bled a lot from a head wound." I watched to see if the mention of blood bothered her. "They've stopped the bleeding, but there's blood all over his head. Right now, they're more worried about broken bones and internal injuries."

I stopped to check her reaction. She only half listened, desperate to get to the other side of those doors. I asked if anyone else was with her. Her neighbor drove her—did she want him to come back to the room with her? "No, my daughter is on the way." I told the visitor assistant to bring the daughter back when she arrived.

We walked back to the room. Mr. Sims was still in CT. The cavernous size of the trauma bay was amplified by absence, the gurney gone and the staff's former activity invisible. I pulled out a chair. She stood for a moment, staring at the place where the bed should be, where her husband had been. I didn't direct her to sit, but when I sat, she followed. It felt like we arrived on the scene just after a disaster, surveying the damage, wondering what we missed. If she had someone with her, I might have left for a moment, to fit in another intervention for a waiting patient, but I couldn't leave her in this desolate place, alone with her dread.

I saw the bag of bloody clothes in the corner. This is usually when I would hand them to the family member so they could go through the pockets for keys, a phone, a wallet, and instruct me on what to toss and what to keep. I would have loved to have a task to distract us from this foreboding quiet. But I didn't want her to see those blood-soaked clothes before she saw her husband. I decided I'd give those to the daughter when she arrived, already placing expectations on her to be calm and capable. Suddenly the silence was broken by the rattle of the gurney approaching, pushed by techs from radiology and the ER, with the nurse behind them. The nurse quickly hooked Mr. Sims back up to the monitors and then turned to us.

I introduced them, and the nurse repeated the general information about Mr. Sims's status. She asked the wife a few questions about his health history. The doctor walked in, rubbing his hands together to work in the white hand-cleansing foam. He saw Mrs. Sims but gave the patient his attention, noting the numbers on the monitors, asking questions of the radiology techs and the nurse. Then he turned to us, bent down, and offered his hand as I introduced them.

The doctor started at the beginning: "What was your husband doing today?" Then he filled in the blanks: "Apparently no one saw him fall, but he was found on the ground with the ladder on its side. We don't know how far he fell, but his head hit hard. He's got a wound there that bled a lot—we'll close that up with sutures. He's broken his right femur—that's the thigh bone—and his right arm. The good news is that we don't see any internal injuries and his vital signs are pretty good, but we'll keep a close eye on him. The big worry is that head injury. We may need to put a tube down his throat to be safe, in case he stops breathing."

Mrs. Sims stared at her husband on the gurney, then turned to the doctor. "Do you think he'll make it?" The doctor was crouching down to be on the same level with Mrs. Sims. He held eye contact. "I do. His numbers look good and he's a pretty healthy fella, but it was a bad fall, and it will take a while to know how serious his head injury was. But we can fix the fractures. He'll get admitted to ICU. Kathryn will keep you posted on that process, and if you have a question for me, let her know."

As he walked out, a wild-eyed woman staggering toward the room looked at him in terror. The visitor assistant walked beside her, tossed a "good luck" look to me before turning back to her desk. This was the daughter, and she was not going to be the calm, capable daughter that I wanted her to be. Not in that moment, at least.

Ignoring her mom, she ran up to the gurney. "Dad, Dad, talk to me!"

The nurse said, "He's not talking yet, but he's doing OK."

She burst into tears. "What's all this blood!" She turned to her mom. "What happened?"

Mrs. Sims, who hadn't even approached the bedside yet, left her chair to comfort her daughter. I came with her. She started to tell the story, but the daughter interrupted hotly: "I've told you not to let him on that roof!"

I got between them. "Let's talk about that later. Your mom just got some information from the doctor that we can share with you."

To me she demanded, "Why haven't you cleaned him up!"

I took a breath. "I know it's hard to see him like this, but we start with the most important things, like X-rays, in case he has a life-threatening injury. Cleaning up the blood and stitching up the wound is the last thing we'll do. He'll be going upstairs to ICU. Let me show you where you can wait . . ."

"I'm not leaving!"

I saw the back of the nurse stiffen. We could confront this head on, explain that yes, if we wanted her to leave the room, she would indeed leave. But there was no need for a power play; it would make things worse for her, worse for her mom, worse for us, and possibly worse for Mr. Sims. "That's fine, but there's a private room around the corner in case you need to use the phone, use the restroom, or take a break."

The daughter dismissively turned away from me. Mrs. Sims agreed to let me show her the Family Room. When we got into the carpeted room with lamps, couches, and soothing artwork, she apologized for her daughter. "She's always been like that, high strung, but she'll calm down. She loves her daddy." I murmured my understanding and made sure she knew how to find her way back to the treatment room. I'd separated his belongings from his bloodied clothing. I showed her both bags. She accepted the belongings and told me to throw the clothes in the trash.

They'd be allowed to come and go as they pleased now, unless a medical intervention like intubation had to occur, or unless the daughter interfered with treatment or kept picking at her mom. I was worried about that, the daughter hurling more blame at her mother, but hoped the mom's presence would have a calming effect, that I wouldn't have to stay with them, intervene, or call Security to escort the daughter out, for everyone's sake.

When staff was uncomfortable with who was in the room, their stress increased. This could result in a rift with the family, which complicated my job and meant that we'd all be on edge for the duration of the visit, with the added inconvenience of a probable official complaint. But worse than discomfort and the overuse of my time and attention was the possible effect on the patient, the risk that a distracted nurse might miss a vein or fail to notice a subtle change in the patient's condition not reflected on the monitor.

I returned to my list of tasks and caught up on new patients. When I checked back on the Sims family, I gave them the room number in ICU, and when they rolled him out of the ER, I took them upstairs to orient them to the ICU area. I modeled how to use the intercom from the waiting room to the ICU nurses' station, telling the secretary who answered that I brought up the Sims family and they'd like to see Mr. Sims as soon as possible. The daughter was upset that she wasn't allowed to follow her dad into the room, but ICU is more restrictive, and they don't have advocates to "manage" family members. I told Mrs. Sims that I'd be thinking of her and her husband, that I hoped he'd have a quick recovery. She thanked me, and I left.

I don't know if Mr. Sims recovered. I could have found out, but a traumatic injury like his happened almost every shift, sometimes more than once. I willed myself to not be curious, overwhelmed by the thoughts of holding them all in my mind or heart. But as I walked down the long maze of ICU corridors, I would say my prayers for them, holding the patient and family in light. Instead of the elevator, I took the stairs, preferring to use the four flights back down to the ER to get ready for the next patient.

Even those who crave the excitement of a trauma never want it to end in death. No one wants the finality of loss to befall anyone. In a place where physical and emotional space is constantly violated, to share a death with a stranger's family is the ultimate intrusion into emotional intimacy. Brought into a family's circle, we are woven into a story that will be told as long as the threads hold. But like so many ER moments unforgettable to patients and families, we find a way to make it routine. What is an exceptional event for them has happened before for us, and will happen again.

Nurses and techs go on to other patients, but the social worker is tethered to the experience for hours. First, we find the family. When they arrive, we stay with them until they leave, or we hand them off to our relief. There are interruptions in our interactions, conversations that must be made with the coroner and organ procurement agency, as the bureaucracy of a death imposes itself on grieving. The process demands a sort of frenetic switching, a toggling from the intense emotions of the family to a phone call reviewing criteria for donation eligibility. It's tempting to anchor ourselves to the business of forms and protocols, to find refuge in those matter-of-fact details. But the family comes first, and they are better served by our not detaching from them too quickly. Routine and rhythm keep our focus on the steps when emotional intensity threatens to engulf us.

All we have to offer the family are small things: a question answered by the doctor, the retrieval of the patient's wedding band, a hand on their arm as they see their loved one dead for the first time.

These are way-finding threads. You unwind them to accompany the family into their maze of grief. The threads are elements of your routine, leading you in and leading you out.

We guide the family into their labyrinth of hell. And then we leave them there. It isn't fair, but after seeing the unfairness of life day after day, we no longer expect fairness.

△

Families do find their way out of that maze of grief, but we don't get to see that. Once in a rare while, you encounter a family you met on that dark day. Out in the sunlight you won't recognize them, but you pretend to, because they definitely remember you.

Sometimes you remeet them inside the ER—they are a patient for something minor, or there as a visitor. Being back overwhelms their

senses, but despite tears, there is a lightness you know wasn't there before. They miss the patient terribly but are surviving. They are getting
through, finding their way: Grief is not a cave; it's a tunnel.

Grief

Grief feels like a cave.
An aimless groping
Into a black, deepening void.
Into your hand I press
The only candle I have,
A message
To flicker in the darkness of your soul:
Grief feels like a cave, but it
Is not a cave.
Grief is a tunnel, a journey.
The blackness is the same.
The only difference is Hope.

—Marilyn Gryte

I never expected to have a favorite grief poem, but then I never
expected to encounter so much death. I first heard it in a grief workshop led by the author, Marilyn Gryte. She was a nurse who worked in
maternal health and then became a licensed professional counselor.

Poems like this are helpful to have on hand when writing bereavement cards, professionally and personally. Because of my work I am
more likely now to offer what I once dismissed as an insignificant gesture. Before I started working in the ER, I only sent such cards to those
closest to me.

Grief is intensely isolating no matter how many loved ones share
that pain. If you've received condolence cards, you were probably surprised by how comforting it was to have others reach out, to recognize
your loss, even in that simple way.

I was part of a multidisciplinary team that created the ER's bereavement outreach program in my second year. If a patient died in the ER, the team sent cards to the next of kin for a year. We included support resources and sometimes poems. Every family got a (nonreligious) card during the Christmas season with an article on getting through the holidays. The group creating the program included the ER nurse educator, the hospital chaplain, and an oncology social worker, who led a community support group for those dealing with grief. Once we started the outreach, the team included ER advocates and ER nurses as well.

For twenty-seven years, part of my holiday to-do list included finding, preparing, and writing cards to dozens of families I knew only through their loved ones' deaths. I'd search for cards illustrating the solace of winter beauty, the "peace of the season," wincing at the plethora of bright cards bursting with excessive cheer. Amid the exuberance of the season, I sat alone with a stack of blank cards beside a stack of postmortem documents, reliving dozens of sad and traumatic experiences, forcing myself to recall the families, envisioning them in their first holiday season without their loved one. Each year a new stack of families, cards, and me, striving to convey something comforting.

Initially I had misgivings about this kind of outreach. Would a card be a painful jolt on what might otherwise be a good day, a day when the recipient woke up not feeling sad? How could a card from a stranger have any meaning? Their loved one died in the ER—on our watch; did they really want to hear from us?

While we were creating our outreach program, I got in touch with local support groups, to better know our resources and to learn from the experts—those working with the bereaved, both as peer counselors and as professionals.

One group I contacted was The Compassionate Friends. Started in England by a chaplain who realized that parents suffering the loss of a child could do more for each other than anything he could offer them, this national organization is run by grieving parents for grieving parents.

Our local chapter allowed me to attend a meeting and graciously gave me feedback about our outreach plans. Each person and situation is different, but they assured me that a bereavement card from someone the family may not recall, or never met at the hospital, is unlikely to offend. A grieving person is living with their loss day in and day out.

A coworker whose young child died told me that she felt worse after the first year. So many people told her the pain would magically ease after a year, as if her grief could be scheduled on the calendar. She had clung to that desperate hope. When after a year her pain didn't ease, she was devastated. The amount of time it takes for grief to grow less acute is different for everyone.

One thing we offered in bereavement outreach was the opportunity to visit the room where we cared for their loved one, the room where they died. A few families took us up on this as a way to connect to the deceased's final moments.

When our bereavement program was about five years old, I heard from Patricia, the wife of a salesman who died in a car accident near our town, two states away from where he and Patricia lived. I'd called Patricia the night it happened. As I'd spoken to her, I'd held his wallet open, gazing at the pictures of her and their two-year-old son. I later sent her follow-up cards. She called me to let me know she planned a memorial trip. Her husband had donated his eyes. Her final stop would be in Atlanta to attend the yearly memorial service held by the organ procurement organization.

She traveled along her husband's last route, staying in the same hotels. She went to the site of the accident, and then she came to meet those of us involved in his care, including me. The day of Patricia's visit, the charge nurse kept that trauma room empty. The nurse who had cared for her husband came in on her off day to sit with us there and answer questions.

We had mailed Patricia his belongings long ago, but I'd kept one thing out—a tiny card tucked into his wallet with the typed names and numbers of friends and family. When we have a patient come in without family, finding a card like that is like discovering gold. It gave me names for those pictures in his wallet and the means to connect with them. I was both grateful and saddened—such treasure is bittersweet.

I handed the card to Patricia. She smiled. "His sister made this when he started traveling so much. We always worried about him." This man's family knew about worst-case scenarios, and if one befell him, they were determined to be found quickly.

The physician took time out between patients to join us. There wasn't much to say, but Patricia seemed to take comfort in putting faces to our names and seeing where her husband had been brought. The ER was no longer just a cold clinical space in her imagination, full of unknown people scurrying from patient to patient. We were real people, caring people.

"Can I take your picture?" Glances between the three of us indicated this was fine, though we all knew this was a first—we'd never posed for such a picture before. She'd toted a small camera into the ER. We stood in the room, me, the nurse, and the doctor, as she stood a few feet back and snapped. I never saw that photo, but I imagine us holding expressions of slightly sad smiles with kind eyes.

Every nurse I ever asked to come to this sort of meeting with a family was willing. I believed that an emotional connection with their work added meaning—the patient was more than a body in which lines and leads were placed, medicines given, and tests administered.

Some nurses alluded to seeking this connection when they agreed to come in and meet with family, but mostly they indicated that this was part of their job as healers: someone needed them, and nurses go where they are needed.

Sometimes the request to visit the patient's room was made by a family member who was present in the ER when their loved one died. Their memories disjointed, they sought clarity, a firmer container for their loss. Usually, a family would make this request within a year of the death, but late in my career, a woman named Amanda made the request three years after her mother's death.

As we walked to the room where Amanda's mother had died, she noted where it was situated within the department. "Oh, this is where the room is! It's right here, next to the others." She sounded surprised, reconciling the actual location with her memory, as if the room stood alone in her mind's eye, apart from the business of the ER, in the same stark way that the experience stood apart for her. Now she saw it was part of a row of trauma rooms, in a hub of activity directly across from the watchful eye of the charge nurse.

In Mark Epstein's book *The Trauma of Everyday Life*, he explains how we hold "absolutisms" about life, trusting that the world is stable and predictable, that children do not die, and parents always survive. When these absolutisms fail, we have a singularity of experience that splits us off from reality. Traumatic experiences "cannot be held in normal memory . . . they never make it into the part of the brain that makes sense of the emotional experience."[1]

Amanda found the room both familiar and strange. We sat, and she told me about her mother. They had been close, but her mom's last year of life was a haze of relentless caregiving. Their relationship had become strained, but at the core, she said, their relationship was loving, full of mutual regard and respect. She showed me a picture of her mom and her at the beach at sunset. Heads together, they were laughing in golden light.

Amanda told me she was reconstructing her memories of her mom, and this was the last piece. She wanted me to know her mom was more than the patient who died on the gurney in that room. I later thought about my father's death. I sat beside him as he died, but now had regrets. Could I have made him more comfortable in those last moments? Could I have made those final weeks more fulfilling, or at least distracted him from the dread of the inevitable?

He loved to laugh more than anyone I've met, but he was always the instigator, telling jokes with convoluted, rambling stories, getting so tickled with anticipation of the punch line that when he finally reached it, he could barely get it out. His performance was funnier than his punch lines.

All out of energy in those last weeks, he would have still appreciated a joke. I wasn't the comedian of the family, and I didn't feel like laughing, but making him laugh again would have been a gift to us both.

---

1. Mark Epstein, *The Trauma of Everyday Life* (Penguin Books, 2014), 53, 148.

△

Even when a patient receives excellent care, if the family does not have positive contact with ER staff, or has an interaction that's harsh, the family feels much less confident about the care their loved one received. This is especially true if that negative interaction is with the physician.

A positive rapport between doctor and family is key to acceptance of an unwanted outcome for the families of patients who received life-saving interventions. Ideally, the doctor meets the family while such efforts are underway and again after the code is called and the patient pronounced dead. But often the patient comes in coding, and the doctor works at the bedside until resuscitation efforts stop. The first time they meet the family is when notifying them of the death.

Every doctor has a personal style of notification, a rhythm, a way to lead themselves into and out of that hardest of conversations. They don't vary it much, if at all. Advocates learn each doctor's style and make adjustments. Some doctors ask the family for the backstory: *"Tell me what was going on today."* But this eases the family into false relief; if the doctor wants to hear all this, then surely the patient is alive and has a chance. Usually, the advocate knows otherwise. When the family would steal a look at me, I would wear a look of resignation and regret, preparing myself for the shock wave when, finally, the doctor spoke the conclusive words that upended their world.

Advocates often vented to each other about this style of notification, frustrated that it prolonged the tension and exacerbated the shock. We wondered why doctors did it—perhaps as an attempt to connect with the family before giving traumatic news. Or perhaps it was genuine curiosity about the patient's condition before arrival, knowing they were unlikely to get that information once the family heard the patient had died. The most likely reason for this method was because they were taught it, either in a class or by example. It had the appeal of giving the doctor time to ease into a public confession of a failed outcome—a stalling technique.

Each time I was absorbed in the family's emotions; I didn't always consider the challenge for the physician, because the family came first. Doctors are professionals. A death may mean they have a bad day, but it's nothing like the family's bad day.

I may have underestimated the difficulty of this duty for physicians. A life ending on their watch may be a personal loss or perceived as a failure to achieve their professional imperative—to save lives. I didn't think of it this way because I saw them doing all they could do to help the patient survive. But an ER director told me about a conversation she'd had with a physician administrator about the necessity of saying "sorry" to the families of patients who die. The physician administrator, mindful of liability, felt that saying sorry implied that the ER had done something wrong or failed to do enough.

This was beyond my comprehension. It was the mid-nineties, and I thought we were well past such mindsets. That physician administrator was maybe in his fifties, about twenty years older than me. The ER director kindly broke it down for him: In these circumstances, his saying sorry wasn't about his work but about connecting with the family in their loss. It was about empathy, not blame. To his credit, he came around. And I learned the phrase "blameless apology."

In later years, the advocates joked that someone new was teaching the death notification class to medical students because younger doctors very consciously included *sorry*, as in, *"I'm sorry for your loss."* Most also knew to include the words *they died*. When instead the physician said, *"They didn't make it,"* or *"There's nothing else we can do,"* a family would sometimes turn to me as the doctor walked out, the thinnest strand of hope bending backward—*"So, she's still alive?"*—and I would have to say words that left no doubt and crushed all hope.

What happened next depended on the family. Sometimes there was a stillness in the room, a momentary calm as the words pushed their way past the natural inability to accept the unacceptable. Sometimes there was no stillness. The reaction was immediate. There could be soft denials, arms flung out to grasp anyone within reach. There were tears, sometimes wailing. The Family Room would become a sinking ship. Chairs and lamps were hurled, fists flew into walls, the door would be thrown open, and someone would run out, leaving the others staggering.

△

No one tells you not to cry. Not at social work school, not in hospital orientation, not in ER training. In fact, they tell you the opposite: Crying means you're human.

When I heard this, I always thought, *Thanks, but no thanks. Crying makes things messy.* The truth is I feel vulnerable when I cry, and I prefer to feel strong and in control, a coping mechanism from my itinerant childhood, when lack of control made me feel persistently unsafe.

The first time I saw the raw sorrow of a family openly expressed, I was stunned. Expressive, intense reactions were not my norm, at least not in regard to grief. My family could be loud in our disagreements and laughter, but our grief was quiet. Not repressed or denied, but there was no sobbing or wailing. Maybe it was the military influence, the sense that such displays would be undignified or weak. Or maybe our family's muffled style was genetic, passed down from grandparents raised in the rural parts of Tennessee and Alabama, stoic acceptance of life's losses without complaint.

I was new to the ER and to this kind of expression, but I knew the worst thing to do would be to try to control how someone mourns. So, I wasn't overly influenced by colleagues' stern looks that implied I needed to subdue this type of reaction. Yes, someone who is wild with anguish might cause safety concerns. Other patients and families need to be considered, but we can make a lot of room for different kinds of grief if we are willing to face our own discomfort.

Allowing patients' families to grieve and allowing yourself as the professional to grieve are two entirely different things. You fear you'll lose control, start sobbing, and be useless; after all, you have a job to do. ER staff learn to rationalize their way out of grief: The patient was driving too fast, or under the influence; they weren't compliant with their meds; they had an unhealthy lifestyle; they were doing something stupid. Anything to keep death distant. The death of a healthy adult or a child undercuts our absolutisms—what we tell ourselves about the world. If a death is senseless, it could happen to you.

Every shift brought something sad. I stifled the reflex to cry over and over until I couldn't cry even outside the ER—whether beside my tearful husband watching *Brokeback Mountain* or at my father's funeral. Nevertheless, the deaths that were among the hardest for me were those when no one visibly grieved. I much preferred wailing to stoicism. Was I gaining some cathartic release from families' lamentations? Maybe. Grieving openly felt more honest, more congruent with what had just happened and less compliant with the ER routine. Death is normalized in the ER, its impact thereby dismissed. Part of me rebelled against being part of a structure that strove to keep death tidy. If I didn't see someone grieve over a body, it was harder for me to move on. If no one else was there for the deceased, I felt like the appointed griever by default. But what good is a mourner-by-proxy who can't even cry?

When crying has left you, you realize why you miss it. It provides a release, a cleansing. You feel better afterward. It makes you feel connected to the world and its woes. When the tears won't come, you feel like a machine.

If crying means you're human, then what does it mean when you can't cry?

The family's response to the patient can trigger an emotional response from staff. Something in the way the son spoke to his mother, the way the husband smoothed her hair, can sneak over staff's emotional barriers and evoke our own connections to loved ones.

When I've seen staff torn up over a death, at most they've shed a few tears or released a single sob when hugged by a coworker. There is nothing wrong with crying, even in front of families. If they notice at all, they are touched that you are touched. Mostly, staff try to keep their emotions in check because no one wants the family to feel they need to comfort us. Still, families often do.

When a family reaches toward you through the fog of their loss, it feels impossibly wrong and indisputably right at the same time. It's not their job. We're the ones expected to be strong for them; comforting staff should be the least of their concerns. They haven't found their footing in this brand-new impossible reality—a world without this person in it. The last thing they should worry about is our feelings. Yet in reaching out to extend us comfort, they bring us into their experience. We lose some of the separateness we maintain with strangers—a wall comes down, and the isolation of grief lessens for us and the family. Amid the overwhelming helplessness we all feel in the face of death, offering comfort is a positive action, a reminder that in such times we retain the power of choosing our response.

I know that the small things we do for families at these times matter because they help us connect to each other. The aide who called me when my mother-in-law died cried as she gave me the news. I soothed her, and her tears comforted me. After my mother-in-law's memorial service, my husband's family filled our house, but a few of my close friends came as well. Their presence was such a meaningful acknowledgment of my loss. My mother took comfort in the gentle way the hospice nurse bathed my father the morning he died. Two of my husband's longtime friends demonstrated their support when they made the four-hour drive for my father's funeral. Every condolence card I received helped me feel less alone.

In being tender with a grieving family, the ER staff constructs an experience that runs parallel to the trauma, contradicting the impossibility of loss and softening the edges of what threatens to tear them apart. We cannot change what has happened, but we can be a reminder that amid terrible loss and sadness there is also kindness. This may cushion the depth of the abyss.

When you walk a family to the outside doors, ensuring they have a safe driver and you have their contact information, they usually thank you. It is confounding. You represent the day that their life fell apart—why would they thank you? But you realize that in their place, you might do the same. They have been through something hard, and you stayed beside them. Perhaps they are simply making an obligatory reflex, a reach toward normalcy.

You try to accept their thanks with grace, you say again how sorry you are, you make your hand available, but if they are going to hug you, it will be now. If they open their arms, you step into them—no matter what your personal rule is about not touching. You say goodbye after spending anywhere from thirty minutes to eight hours together, unlikely to see each other again after sharing one of the most emotional experiences of their lives.

They leave the hospital, but they do not leave your thoughts. You think of them the rest of your shift and the next day when you wake up, knowing they awoke to a strange new reality. That they are making decisions about the funeral, dealing with whatever is left behind, physically and emotionally, and—most difficult—telling others, spreading the strange new reality into their world.

△

When someone I know dies, I am vividly aware of my mental conflict, the cerebral gymnastics required for acceptance of loss. I can't wrap my head around it.

Child psychologist Jean Piaget defined the concept of object permanence, or the understanding that a hidden object still exists.[2] His studies showed that most of us have object permanence at least by eight months of age. This explains why younger infants delight in playing peekaboo. Until the infant has object permanence, someone who appears gone is, to them, really gone. Their sudden return is pure magic. Then we learn object permanence and regard the world differently for the rest of our years. Death requires us to unlearn this early lesson. Our person is gone and is never coming back.

Even as I grieve a loss, I marvel at my brain's bewilderment, as if there is something of the wild in us yet. Humans have always lost loved ones. After all these thousands of years, it seems like our brains would have developed some capacity or synapse to reconcile a new absence. Faith helps some and time helps almost all, but I wonder about

2. Jean Piaget, *The Construction of Reality in the Child*, translated by M. Cook (Basic Books, 1954).

physiological change. Part of me likes that we have not outsourced grief, found a way to bypass the experience. For all our fancy inventions, we have old-fashioned hearts.

Do It Our Way

When you make the difficult decision to ask for help, you probably know what you want that help to look like. You have certain expectations based on your experience living your life; you know what works and what doesn't. When help comes wrapped up in a different shape, you may look at it and wonder if it's worth the bother of accepting—is it going to make any difference at all?

You are the expert of your life, but as a patient in a medical setting, you are suddenly demoted from CEO to intern—*"We know what's best. You have problems, and we have the answers and the resources, or the keys to accessing them. You have only to trust us, listen to us, and do exactly what we say."*

Most patients know this is the setup when they walk through the doors. They need help, and they want to be perceived as reasonable, positive, and likable. If a patient likes us and believes we like them, rapport blossoms. It is this need to be agreeable that sparks the "Yes, but." The patient is struggling to be both compliant and honest, but if being honest means telling us why they cannot comply with our advice, we don't want to hear it.

In the ER, respect for self-determination is trumped by absolute medical truths: If you continue to abuse alcohol, your diabetes will kill you; a heart attack is coming unless you change your lifestyle; if you don't stay on your blood pressure medicine, you'll have a stroke; what we found on the CT scan could be lethal, so you must have more tests.

If we find something that is trying to kill you, it's the doctor's job to let you know. It's a social worker's job to support and motivate you, to find a way toward a manageable plan, all without delaying discharge from the ER—because, remember, the patient who is waiting for a room is the patient in the most danger, and there is always a patient waiting even when there's not. It's a mindset.

Medical people are stubbornly focused on applying medical truths indiscriminately. Nothing short of absolute compliance will appease them. Patients who return with the same problem, possibly made worse by time, are judged by their degree of compliance.

I grew to hate that word: *compliance*. It is a subjective label disguised as an objective medical term. If you did not comply, you did not follow the rules, so of course you did not get better. The label of noncompliance is given without regard for a patient's intention, ability, or resources (like not having a car or insurance). The details ("excuses") are dismissed, and the patient is blamed, partly to relieve the provider's psyche, because all these failures take a toll. Noncompliance means the patient is at fault.

The confluence of individual, social, and medical system failures occurs in the ER and produces an ever-flowing waterfall that pounds you down and obscures the successes in a mist. The patients who survive, who make changes, who get the help they need—those patients don't come back. They are not part of your landscape. At most you have moments of hope based on brief interactions—a trauma patient or a resuscitated patient makes it from the ER to ICU. But medical professionals know the odds are against those patients. If the patient rolled out of the ER alive, it's not a failure, but is it a success?

In the medical world the patient is the default scapegoat. This was contrary to my education and training. Social work teaches you to see how social factors contribute to a person's challenges, how they act on the person, influence them, and limit their options. I thought of clients or patients as victims of their circumstances. ER culture rejects this view, insisting on personal responsibility even when a dire social situation crashes into the extensive needs of a medical condition. I tried to stay aware of this tendency, but even now in retirement, I see it took root. I recently saw a wrecked car sitting in a ditch, on a road I regularly drive. I instantly thought, *That's what happens when you drive drunk,* with a wave of disgust, before my second thought: *It could have been a deer.* Yes, the driver might have swerved to avoid something in the road, as we all would. Something like this could happen to any of us.

△

Paula was a diabetic who abused alcohol. I met her in my early days at the ER, again and again. We would give her fluids, test her sugar, lecture her about care for her diabetes, and get her a ride home. Because she was making return trips related to alcoholism, she sometimes saw our mental health counselor. She was my age—twenty-eight.

Admissions to mental health or alcohol/drug detox programs are difficult to obtain. Priority is given if you have the insurance, have the motivation to go voluntarily, or seem to be a significant risk to yourself or someone else. None of that applied to Paula.

She wanted to go home from the moment she arrived. She was never the one who had called the ambulances that brought her; someone else would make that call when she passed out. No one ever came in with her, so we had no idea who the caller was. But Paula always had a number to call for a ride home, and they always came.

It would take a few hours to get her sober and stable enough to discharge, and during that time she would try to leave, despite wearing only a hospital gown and being hooked up to an IV. She required some watching, which was a nuisance for busy staff, yet no one expressed dislike for her, maybe because she wasn't overtly hostile or combative, or maybe because she didn't bother feigning remorse.

Paula didn't apologize and didn't ask for anything except to go home. She didn't even bother with "Yes, but." She was silent, her eyes a cold stare as we gave her the numbers to call for mental health and diabetic follow-up.

She didn't ask for our help. Like most of my peers, I was not surprised when she was not compliant, but unlike most of my peers, I didn't consider her wholly responsible for her diabetes, her alcoholism, or her noncompliance.

Land of the Jinx

In the ER, the word *quiet* is taboo. It cannot be spoken by anyone working in the ER. Instead, we say, "The Q word." Any hospital employee, even one just passing through who notes an empty waiting room or a cluster of open patient rooms, will be met with scowls if they remark, "It's quiet!" They've jinxed us. They'll be blamed for the next trauma that rolls in, and all the subsequent ones until they get off shift. They won't make that mistake again.

ER workers are superstitious. So are the medics. Probably firefighters and police are as well. Frontline workers face the relentlessness of life's chaos. Lives can be turned upside down in seconds, our sense of control whisked right out from under us.

I knew paramedics who rode motorcycles without a helmet or didn't wear seat belts. They no longer believed that death could be cheated, delayed, or prevented—if it's your time, it's your time. So, all those people they worked on who died? It was their time. Fatalistic worldview serving as protective adaptation, a way to keep working and living without the fear taking over.

But workaday destiny seemed to be something else, something you could influence by what you did and did not do. According to ER culture, you will jinx your current good luck if you remark on it. When working a calm shift, if the charge nurse is asked how their day is going, the only safe response is "It's been nice."

There's also a little dance around words to avoid implying that we desire the shift to go a certain way. As if a mischievous universe is eavesdropping so it can conjure up the opposite.

Running in the background of our vulnerable minds seems to be a belief or a spark of hope that if we can pinpoint the part we play in bad things happening, we can change our future through our behavior and keep those bad things at bay.

We've seen the worst of what the universe can dish out. We have to believe we have some means of mitigating not only a rough shift at work but the odds of a worst-case scenario happening to us. If it's not accommodating superstitions, maybe prayer, a belief in things happening for a reason, or a set of rules to live by will spare us from the deadly car accident, the devastating illness, the violent assault. Anything to avoid the fact of our constant vulnerability—because who can live with that?

Even if you avoid jinxes, you can be labeled a "shit magnet." This title is earned when, while working on a day when all hell breaks loose, someone recalls that you were also there the last time all hell broke loose. This label is especially likely if you were in the same role both days—charge nurse, trauma nurse, or triage nurse.

Often the bad luck is ascribed to pairs working together, coworker combos that seem to synergize havoc that impacts the entire department. Assignments are sometimes changed for no other reason than "when Amanda works on the same pod with Carrie, the nicest day goes to shit."

There is always someone looking to blame someone else for a hard shift, to point a finger at you before you point a finger at them. There is something in human nature that demands a scapegoat.

Not everyone minds the moniker of shit magnet. Some wear it proudly, like a superpower they threaten to pull out at will to wreak havoc. The ability to shape the day is empowering. Who wouldn't choose this over helplessness?

$$\triangle$$

When a patient we're accustomed to seeing frequently has not been seen in the ER for some time, we must not say their name. Speaking their name will cause them to arrive. If the patient appears within two weeks of saying their name, your violation of this rule will be recalled.

Jeff, a nurse tech, had only worked in the ER for a few weeks, but he'd already met Arnold three times. Jeff leaned on the counter of the nurses' station and casually mentioned that every Friday night that he worked, Arnold had come in. This was Friday night. We pelted Jeff with groans and glares, and when Arnold came in a few hours later, Jeff was in big trouble.

Arnold was an alcoholic in his sixties. He came in full of spit and venom, cursing the staff and threatening to punch us. Seen downtown weaving, falling, or ranting, a Good Samaritan would call the ambulance. Seeing the medics, Arnold would erupt in fury. The medics didn't want to bring him in, but turning away from someone in need—even if that person is raging at you—is not a good look for a community provider. If you want to refuse ambulance transportation, you have to be able to demonstrate that you're competent to make that decision. Arnold's frenetic resistance only made him seem more in need of medical services.

They'd wrangle him onto a stretcher, strap him down, and bring him to us. Once in our doors, we were obligated to assess him and provide the needed care. The doctor would cajole him enough to get a basic assessment, and if his vital signs were stable, he'd be released. If his alcohol level was too high, he would stay awhile, receive fluids if an IV was possible. Appropriately, on this visit, Jeff was assigned to be his nurse tech.

Once ready for discharge, Arnold became my problem. He never had anyone to call but often had a place to go, which he would share only after unleashing a torrent of obscenities. We'd call a cab and keep him in his room until they arrived, to avoid exposing other patients to his tirades. Security would escort him out and into the cab. He might be back the next month, the next day, or even a few hours later. A visit from Arnold impacted the entire department. I never heard Jeff mention his name again.

The patients whose absence we notice are the patients that stand out. They may be difficult to care for medically or behaviorally. They may be rude, violent, exceedingly sweet, or outrageously funny. They scream obscenities, sing to us, or play a harmonica; they have interesting tattoos or scars; they bring a daughter or a pimp in with them who drives us crazy.

They come to us lonely, hurting, or scared. Some use the ambulance as a medical Uber to this part of town and fabricate a reason to be seen. Sometimes they're in a long battle with drugs or alcohol. Their absence could mean they're doing better, but we assume the worst.

We whisper our theories to a trusted coworker about what's become of them—not wanting others to hear us saying the name. We shrug away any guilt of bestowing worst-case scenarios on them. In the Land of the Jinx, we protect the absent patient by not speaking our best wishes for them. We protect the current patients by having no room numbered thirteen.

ER room numbering can be confusing and seem random, but omitting thirteen is intentional. In both our old ER and the new one, the decision was made for rooms to go from twelve to fourteen. Staff does not want to care for a patient in room thirteen, and upon entering it, a patient will become convinced that this is a worst-case scenario on top of a worst-case scenario.

△

I've never felt especially lucky. When my brother and I argued over something, like who got to sit in the front seat of the car, my dad flipped a coin. Being younger, I always got to choose first, and I always called "heads," mostly because that side was more visually appealing (what even is that image on "tails"?). My brother always won. I don't recall a single time when the coin landed on heads, but I was sure that it would as soon as I called tails. Maybe that's why I don't court luck—it was never there for me.

One time when the ER was slammed, with every room taken, ambulances coming in, and the waiting room so backed up that urgent patients were waiting more than two hours and nonurgent patients more than four, I was feeling my oats. Comfortable in my role and with the staff on shift, I leaned over to the charge nurse and devilishly said, "Well, at least it can't get any worse." She aimed laser eyes at me, but I chuckled. We both knew that it could always get worse. But if we did fall into a pit of hell on that shift, we managed to climb out, as always.

I dismissed luck and jinxes as too randomly superstitious, but I am a sky watcher, and I note the cycles of the moon. I want to believe that a full moon influences our experiences. On a busy night shift, someone will ask if the moon is full, and if it is, they seem vindicated—they have found their scapegoat, a reason for the mayhem. But my perception was that we seemed just as likely to have a slow night on a full moon as a busy one. I read studies that indicated there was no correlation. I grew annoyed at my coworkers' lunar accusations throughout the entire shift. I'd given up trying to find a pattern to the chaos of the ER, and I wanted company in my rejection of order in favor of a random universe theory.

In contrast to the patients in the ER, I realized I was very lucky. I didn't ask for luck's blessings . . . or perhaps I did, as I lay in bed, praying for my loved ones' protection. Who was I praying to? I no longer knew.

I didn't buy into the full moon connection, but when the thirteenth falls on a Friday, that's an ER shit show for real.

The Business of Helping

When I went through graduate school in social work, there were two tracks, clinical or organizational. I chose organizational because I wanted to help shape entities that were saving the world, preferably feeding children in developing countries. I wanted to be part of a big organization with a big plan.

As a social worker, especially when starting out, you need to have that desire to save the world—though you keep that desire secret because it makes you look naive. If you don't have that much heart at the start, you'll not find the courage to brave the dark places where your work is waiting. But if you have too much heart, you'll be crushed, and, even worse, ineffective. You must learn how to not "let your helping get in the way of *helping*."

My undergraduate professor who used this line looked like a scholarly Andy Griffith with fading ginger hair. He said it in his soft North Carolina twang, and I still hear him whenever I find myself getting in the way: when I have an agenda, when I have biases, when I make assumptions—in other words, all the time. Your only hope as a social worker is to achieve enough self-awareness to thwart your worst best intentions.

For example, when a patient is a no-show for a rare slot at a free clinic—the clinic where they could see a physician specialist who volunteers only a few hours a week, which you got them by begging the clinic director—you don't waste time blaming them. Patients have a hard time getting to appointments: transportation issues, long hours at jobs they can't risk losing, lack of childcare, or being too sick that

day even to seek the help they need. When the clinic director calls
to complain that this priceless favor they granted "your patient" was
wasted, you know you'll go out on that limb again, but not for this
patient. Your desire to help them must not undermine your efforts for
the next one. There's always a next one, and maybe the next one will
show up for that coveted appointment.

△

A graduate social work degree qualifies you for a wide array of positions. Any statements I make about exactly what social workers do will
not be accurate. Many social workers are therapists and counselors,
but generally the profession tends to be oriented toward assessment
and problem-solving. In the hospital setting, this may include making plans for discharge: setting up transportation and lining up home
health care or oxygen, finding the cheapest way to get them an essential medication, or finding them an alternative place to go—a domestic
violence shelter, an extended stay hotel, a care facility.

When I joined the ER team, I understood that I signed up for their
mission of improving health and saving lives—a big plan in a pretty
big organization. I knew that my mission within the organization was
unique. While medical staff focused on the "what" of an illness, I focused on the "why." Why was this patient hurt or not getting better?

This line of inquiry is in conflict with the medical mission of ERs.
With their Band-Aid approach to medical care, they can and do save
lives, but once they determine your life is not in immediate danger,
they generally do as little as possible, affixing the tiniest of Band-Aids.
If they're bogged down by investigating the cause of your belly or back
pain, care may be delayed for the patient who's at risk of dying today.
The social work that happens in the ER is a Band-Aid approach as well.
It is the briefest of brief interventional help and assessment.

Some social workers have the same clients for years, but I never
wanted to be a counselor, or have an assigned caseload at a county services department. Although those are essential positions that I value,
that work seemed tedious to me, and the rewards slow in coming,

dependent on the improbability of individuals changing. I wanted more immediate, tangible gratification and a variety of tasks. I also wanted to be part of an organization that worked within a web of organizations in a community. I thought every shift in the ER would bring new patients with new problems, leading me to find new resources. The mission to help would succeed by teamwork.

I thought there would be wider variation in the types of problems to solve, because I expected a larger variety of patients. Anyone can have an accident, I thought, but even accidents are not as randomly distributed as I once believed. Income is a protective factor. A better income gets you a safer car and newer tires. It gets you a safer home, a better diet, and preventative care. It gets you the best follow-up care or gives you choices for a mental health facility or nursing home. Living in an affluent area might mean you have access to a better medical facility. Income and privilege decrease the risk of coming to the ER.

Many patients in the ER are often on the edge or have just fallen off it. They can be desperate, conflicted, flawed . . . human. Everyone who comes to the ER needs resources, even the wealthy. It's an excellent place to have social workers.

$$\triangle$$

Empathy begins before you develop rapport with a patient, fueled by an intent of unconditional positive regard as you walk into the room. Your help doesn't depend on liking them or being able to personally relate to their situation. As we listen closely to their circumstances, we use imagination to fuel our empathy. We set ourselves in the situation to get a visceral feel for their experience. We can pivot into the other person's point of view—see and feel it through their perspective, their belief system, their delusions. Social workers don't always get to be the nice guys. But if we've found a way to *meet the patient where they are*, they sense that we're there to help. Even so, they may examine our offer and find that our variety of help does not match what they were looking for. It's best if, when you first meet them, you don't have a high-stakes hidden agenda crouching behind your smile.

The doctor has two patients in one room, a woman and her teen-age daughter. He tells them the bad news: They both have an STD—the same type of STD. What he doesn't tell them is that he's worried the mom's boyfriend has had sex with the daughter. He asks me to "assess this," which is code for evaluate this concern (without telling them the doctor's suspicions), and when they deny having sex with the same man, determine whether they are lying. If I had met them before the doctor gave them this news, they might not be as guarded, might have dropped their facades and let me see the impact of this diagnosis. But I didn't meet them earlier, and now I enter the room as a doctor's appointee with a specific task. It's more honest to be up front with my intention, but it's less likely to yield honesty from them—people rarely tell a hard truth straight up, especially to an official-seeming stranger.

Alone with the daughter, I come in sideways: "So, you're going to need to tell the guy you had sex with about this, because he needs treatment also." She nods. "Is that going to be hard?"

"No."

"Is it someone you've been seeing for a while?"

"Yeah."

I need more, so I adjust course. "Because of your age, I need to ask—is this a safe relationship?" She looks at me blankly. "Is this some-one you want to have sex with?"

She rolls her eyes. "Yes!" She says it with sarcasm, as if implying she could ever be a victim is a deep insult. After all, she isn't a child, she's *sixteen*!

"Is he your age?"

"He's one year older." Daring me to judge her.

I smile to acknowledge my idiocy. "OK, good, I just had to ask. If there's anything about the situation that you want to tell us, ask for me. My name's Kathryn."

She nods again, this time with an "as if" sneer.

Was she lying? I can't know for sure. Detecting lies is one of those magical qualities I'm supposed to have, and when the patient is vulner-able to harm, I desperately wished for that power. I provided a private place for our conversation, asked the question, and got the answer I needed. Possibly my empathy got in the way, made me want to align with the patient, believe what they told me. I suspect I only sussed out the very worst liars.

Of course medical care must be the primary focus of ERs, but if you're at risk for abuse by someone you live with, that issue may be more pressing than your medical ailment. It seems like this would be common ground, where health and safety overlap, and social workers, medical staff, and patients could all agree on priorities, and often they do. But consider your own priorities: What are you putting before your yearly physical, your overdue colonoscopy? Perhaps you're not taking prescribed medication because of the side effects, or because buying it means you'll be late on the rent. Your reasons don't matter much to your medical team—you're simply noncompliant.

The eighty-year-old woman who lives alone with three dogs won't agree to be admitted for overnight cardiac monitoring followed by a morning stress test. She has to go home to feed those dogs. When a patient is a caregiver, they often put that responsibility first, whether they're caring for a child, an elderly spouse, or a pet.

If a patient refuses admission, an advocate goes in to try to figure out why, with the agenda of convincing them. But persuasion is more likely when you pair it with understanding. If you uncover the reason for their refusal, you honor it, and search for an acceptable solution. This is how you meet a patient where they are instead of imposing your perspective, blind to their situation, concerns, values.

The medical issues can be cut-and-dried to medical staff—if you need to stay for the benefit of your health, you stay. Violating this simple logic can be perceived as an affront, as being willfully noncompliant. But only the patient knows what's going to fall apart if they don't get back home today. And if you don't care enough to acknowledge their biggest concern, why should they trust you with their health?

When I started, I had the aggressive defensiveness of an underdog with the medical staff, fighting for the wishes of the patients and their families. This could be in regard to tests, communication, and even for visiting in the room, as the default was to keep families out. But with time, procedures changed, the advocate role grew, and I personally earned more credibility. As I became a senior staff person in tenure and in age, I felt respected, able to influence individual situations as well as initiate new ways of doing things. I no longer had to fight so hard.

For the social worker, there is no objective "fix it" mission—some body part or disease that needs treatment or further study, separated from the considerations of personality, mental health, social inequities, or poverty. We have the luxury of widening our view to include the person's situation because usually what we do, or fail to do, will not kill anyone—and that is a huge perk.

△

For many people, the ER is the best option for almost any issue: It's always open, and patients will be seen regardless of their ability to pay. But our Band-Aids are often inadequate, and the patients return the next month with the same problem.

A few times we learned we hadn't seen a "frequent flyer" in a while because they were in prison or had died. Death is not usually a desirable outcome, but prison has potential advantages: shelter, mental health services, supervised medication, reduction of access to addictive substances (we hope). Why is imprisonment required to access a safety net of services? Incarceration is neither safe nor desirable, but prisons seem to be used the same way we use hospitals—inappropriately and far too often.

If a frequent-use patient got admitted, advocates in the ER would alert the social workers on the floor, hoping they'd have time to press on a better bandage. And they often did, despite also being under constant pressure to empty rooms. But usually, our frequent-use patients were not admitted; they were discharged from the ER. And if their circumstances improved significantly, it was because someone at another organization took the time to find a longer-term solution: A nurse in the indigent clinic got a patient set up with free medications; an alcoholic patient in rehab got connected to low-cost housing. These organizations weren't bigger with better plans, but they had the one thing we never had—time.

Playing the Odds

Most of my fears involve being trapped. If I'm in a high place, my fear is called acrophobia; if I'm in water, aquaphobia; if I'm in an MRI machine, it's claustrophobia. All these fears are exacerbated by a sense of helplessness—situations I can't control.

Airplane travel combines being stuck with height, motion, and loss of control. It's an experience I wobble through, start to finish. Yet I keep flying, even by myself, even overseas. I tell myself that fear will not stop me from doing anything I truly want or need to do.

Until my children were in their twenties, my fear for them took center stage. That fear was pungent, immediate, and relentless, but now I have to remind myself to worry about them.

I expected to have less fear as I got older, just as I expected more poise and confidence would be bestowed on me—a gift of the birthday milestone fairy. I'd have liked to have fully accepted my body by age forty, to have no qualms speaking my mind by age fifty, and to be free of fear by age sixty. By age seventy I expect wisdom to wrap around me like a soft shawl.

I'd never been afraid of driving or car accidents until my late twenties, just before I started working in the ER. As I drove around with my two young children in our used, hail-dinged minivan, a very specific fear grew.

Our town's bypass has bridges over a river that winds through and around the city. There were several accidents in which the bridge railings collapsed when hit by cars, and those cars plunged into the river. In some cases, the occupants drowned.

The impact alone could kill you, but what terrified me was imagining being trapped in that van with my children, the river closing over us, and only me to get us out alive. I bypassed the bypass.

But I knew avoidance gave power to the fear, and finding alternative routes was complicating my life, so I told my husband. He didn't ridicule or rationalize; he gave me information and a tool. He explained how our vehicle would sink, given its weight distribution, and the best way to get out of the vehicle. He gave me an awl to break a window.

The bridges got fixed, but I always have a window breaker in my car, and thanks to a nurse friend, trauma shears to cut my seat belt.

Death by car is common but varied. For a while I was flummoxed by ejections—people thrown out of their car. I envisioned all these people driving around with their windows wide open. I couldn't fathom a force that would propel someone through the windshield, or that so many people did not wear seat belts. Flying through glass at that speed, your body stopping only when it hits something, results in terrible injuries or death. Wear your seat belt.

By nature, my husband is more safety conscious than I am, and he came to our marriage more experienced with babies due to having five older brothers who all had kids. Other than my fear of bypass bridges, I was the less vigilant parent in terms of general risk awareness, despite my phobias. (By definition phobias are irrational. Rationally I knew flying was safe, for example, so I didn't fear it for my children; I just personally abhorred the sensation of hanging in the air.) When we disagreed about the safety of a situation, we agreed to defer to the parent with the concern.

This meant our kids wore life jackets when toddling around a pier on a lake, or around the edge of a pool, because although we're both good swimmers, he knew it only took a second to sink. He convinced me to keep the pitcher of hot tea far from the counter's edge. When I said, "They've never reached up to pull anything off the counter," he said, "That's not how safety works." He proposed that we never let our kids drink from our glasses, to lessen the chance of burns from their grabbing our mugs of hot coffee while they cuddled on our laps during

those too-early mornings when our reaction times were caffeine defi-
cient. He kept all of us safe.

After I had worked in the ER for a while, that dynamic—safe parent versus sort of clueless parent—began to shift. At that time my kids
were four and five, and I began to see danger everywhere. Cars were
the most frightening because fatal accidents were so common. Driving
is the most dangerous activity that we all engage in routinely, yet we
manage to dismiss it daily.

Once, on a car trip, my kids spied lollipops in the console. They
asked for them, and I handed them over with the caveat that they hold
them out of their mouths when we went over bridges, because if we
were in an accident, it could get lodged in their throats. My husband
gave me a look. He told them to just enjoy the suckers.

I was confused. Clearly this situation was full of obvious dangers: suckers, a known choking hazard; cars, dangerous daily activity
number one; and bridges, my old nemeses. Together, they added up
to a threat I thought I could mitigate only if my children could time
sucking between bridges. In my mind this was totally logical; this was
being safe. A water escape from a vehicle I could manage, but add in
the complexity of choking on a sucker, and all bets were off.

Pointing out that it was statistically unlikely that we would have an
accident while on a bridge as our kids sucked on lollipops, my husband
gently let me know that maybe I'd gone a little off the deep end in my
new awareness of risk. I didn't see it, and I certainly didn't feel it, but I
decided to trust him.

He appreciated that he no longer had to convince me of safety
concerns, but this was a new problem he'd not anticipated—that I
perceived dangers as a frantic game of Whac-A-Mole. With my fears
all over the place, I realized I could infect our kids with loopy logic,
undermine their security, and hinder their ability to accurately assess
danger for themselves.

Some things I was learning in the ER could help our family, so my
husband helped me integrate and use that new information. He set this
up one evening after the kids were in bed. We sat on the threadbare

couch of our rental house. Tiptoeing around my defensiveness by respecting my fear, not ridiculing it, he reminded me of what I knew:
how safety conscious he was. If there was a risk he didn't perceive, he
wanted to know. But he pointed out the emotional intensity of how I
encountered this infusion of new risks—I was being schooled in the
land of worst-case scenarios. I could use him as a harbor from that
land, to sort out what risks were relevant to our family. I agreed, believing that he could assess risks more clearly because he wasn't seeing
the carnage firsthand. He didn't have the sensory overload of seeing
people hurt and sometimes killed on an almost daily basis. We had to
change our old agreement of defaulting to the parent with the safety
concern, because my work environment was changing me. I didn't
work in the real world—I worked in the ER, and the warped perspective it generated was leaking into my homelife.

My kids grew out of their car seats and became reliable seat belt
users, reminding older family members when they forgot or delayed
buckling up. We adopted a catchphrase in our family, mimicking my
father's Southern-accented impression of our daughter, who at four
years old told him, "Fasten your seat belt, honey."

As the kids grew up and out of our sphere of control, I would use
the latest car-crash injury I'd seen to hammer home the horrid consequences of driving under the influence of alcohol or not buckling
up. They nodded their heads wearily at this dramatic litany but eventually got annoyed. "Do you really think we don't get it?" they would
demand, offended. "Do you really think we don't wear our seat belts all
the time?"

I really had no idea. I knew that thinking you know for sure what
your kids do when you're not around was delusional. I knew that seat
belt use wasn't so vigorously consistent when I was growing up. Had
the times changed so much that this safety measure was a given? Could
I trust other parents? Could I trust my kids? I had no real control over
this; I could only nag and pray.

Everyone working in the ER worries that they'll walk into a trauma
room and see their child on the gurney. When a medic calls the charge
nurse with a report from the scene of a car accident, those who are

parents with teens lean over to listen in on the details, desperate to rule out their child as their next patient.

△

In those child-rearing years, I found another by-product of parent-hood was a new directive to keep myself alive. I had to be alive to pro-tect them and to raise them to an adulthood that wouldn't feature the wound of a missing parent. Plus, I liked them; I wanted to hang around and see them grow up.

My imagination was laden with death scenarios, with my husband or me sacrificing our life if it would increase the chance of the other surviving, ensuring our children had at least one parent. In the sinking ship scenario, I take the plunge à la Jack in the movie *Titanic*. After all, in a lifeboat, my kids would need their dad's ingenuity and resilience. Plus, he's boat smart.

After working in the ER for about twelve years, I drove to Atlanta for a workshop in a hard rain one winter day. On the four-lane high-way, I got sandwiched between big rig trucks. I couldn't pull out; I couldn't safely pull over—I was stuck. I clutched the steering wheel, squinting to see the truck in front of me through the frenzied spray of water shooting up from its tires, struggling to keep my eye on it and not steal glances in the mirror at the massive truck right on my tail, or the one rolling up in the lane next to me. Everyone was going too fast for conditions, including me.

After ejections, car crashes with big trucks are the most disturb-ing. In car versus truck, truck wins every time. It doesn't matter how savvy a driver you are. They are too big to stop fast or maneuver. Any dicey driving situation—fog, an unexpected slowdown, driving fatigue or distraction, darkness, wet roads, a hard rain—gets riskier when there's a big truck around. If your paths collide at high speed, the car will be demolished, the driver and passengers possibly killed instantly or trapped until medics pull out whatever is left of them.

I am speaking through the lens of worst-case scenarios—my wheelhouse. Maybe there are fender benders with big trucks, accidents so minor that no one comes to the ER. If those stories exist, I never witnessed them. They cannot be added to my mental mix to dilute the slurry of mangled metal and bodies.

I'm not blaming the truck drivers. I've worked plenty of accidents in which the car driver was at fault. We all make mistakes, but when a big truck is involved, the penalty is higher. I've stood in the room as medics detailed the "mechanism of injury" to help medical staff understand how the body lying before us came to be so broken.

They share what they were told or pieced together, about how the collision occurred, the damage to the vehicles. They describe what they found, the intrusion of the car into the body, how the body was extracted from the rubble.

Driving into Atlanta (there is no rail transport from my town) guarantees being up close to big trucks at high speeds for long stretches of time. I get around them when I can, but when one stays on my tail, or they're too numerous to avoid, I feel the panic rising.

I got to that workshop intact. I was shaken, but there had been no accident, just a whole lot of adrenaline surging through my body. Days later, driving at slowish speeds in my midsize town, the same feeling hit me, even with no trucks or danger in sight.

Those flimsy bypass bridges had been replaced long ago. I drove over them now with nary a concern. The symptoms came at odd times, starting with a feeling of dizziness, which seemed to be triggered by a high speed, making it hard to go the speed limit. But also if I was stopped at a traffic light or boxed in by trucks, I'd be overwhelmed by a feeling of being trapped, certain I would pass out if I couldn't move. My brain was quick to remind me that it had a history of making me pass out—what was to keep me from that now? I'd keep water handy to sip on, the colder the better. The radio sometimes helped, but sometimes made it worse. My heart pounded, and I had to force my breathing to slow down. There were roads where I regularly experienced these symptoms, so I avoided them.

I believe my random driving fears are linked to that rainy day with the trucks because that experience stands out. I've been in car accidents, though no big ones, and none of my fear in those accidents compares to the fear I felt the day of that workshop. My husband said that it's like having all the lingering effects of an accident without ever having the actual accident, my own brand of PTSD, fueled by my imagination. But those sparks had been stoked by the ER. All those car crashes—almost every shift, for years—whittled down my powers of denial. I no longer believed that crashes were unlikely, something that happened to other people.

I continued to drive, but the weirdness didn't completely go away. One friend in the medical field thought this could be a neurological problem. The idea of seeing a neurologist about this was too embarrassing. There is so much shame around our bodies and minds acting in ways we feel are strange. I figured that if it was a medical problem, I'd have further symptoms.

Once when having lunch with my boss outside of work, she mentioned driving in Atlanta, so I told her about this new experience. She used my nickname, the one she gave me: "KK, it sounds like anxiety." She was the first to say this to me.

"But I've always driven to Atlanta. I commuted there daily for months! I'm not afraid of driving." Although I convinced her, I had a seed of doubt—was this "just" a panic attack?

A panic attack feels like you're dying, but I saw that some staff sneered when a patient's medical issue was revealed as "just" anxiety. Patients with panic attacks tend to come in hyperventilating, or worse, with chest palpitations or syncope, which sends staff scurrying to prepare to deliver lifesaving measures. Because staff initially believed there was a real threat to the patient, when anxiety was revealed to be the culprit, they felt played. These patients were dismissed as histrionic and a major waste of time, diverting resources from "real" patients who needed real care.

Even as I denied that I shared this affliction, I looked closer at patients we saw for anxiety. I observed interactions and noticed more nuance. It helped if the patient mentioned their history of panic attacks up front, or, if this was a new experience, if they were open to the idea that it could be anxiety when diagnostic tests came back negative. If the nurse had personal experience with anxiety and understood its confounding nature, they showed more empathy.

Given the many people I knew who were on antianxiety medication, I was sure that mentioning it to my primary care nurse practitioner would result in a prescription. But after we spoke for a while, she encouraged me to keep up my medicine-free approach unless it got worse.

I was surprised. This was contrary to the quick-fix approach I expected from medicine. It seems unusual in our culture to admit to such a problem and not receive a pill. If she didn't think I needed a prescription, then maybe I was being dramatic. Maybe my symptoms weren't that significant, or I'd been overly influenced by coworkers who had no medication hesitancy when it came to self-care, or more likely, I just underplayed the extent of my difficulty.

In other times in my life when my inner turmoil invaded my outer reality, I saw a therapist. The first time was while I was an undergraduate student. A counselor at our college spoke in my psychology class. I liked her warmth and humor. She had a social work degree. She invited us to sample the free counseling services at the college. I hoped that in having her as a therapist, she could serve as a model for me and strengthen my insight into myself. I was also a few months from getting married—and more uncertain about the relationship than I would admit to myself. But I knew that this step was a big one and would be stressful. I saw her on a regular basis until I graduated.

I later joined a Gestalt therapy group. This was experiential learning, vastly more helpful than any class or textbook. When I left that first husband, I saw another therapist for a short time, mostly to grieve the hard lesson that love is not always enough.

Nearing forty, I found a Jungian therapist to help me sort out my vivid sleepwalking dreams. She diagnosed me with mild anxiety, but explained that such a diagnosis was necessary to get insurance to kick in. (The driving incident had not yet happened at this point.) We worked with archetypes of the psyche, and I learned how to understand and respect what my deeper self needed. I recommitted to my creative life, resisting giving everything of myself away to my family or my job. I saw this therapist regularly for over two years and expected to have her as a longtime counselor, but she died unexpectedly. She was a tremendous resource that I'd invested in, pouring my life stories out for her. She made sense of those stories, helping me voice them and listen to new ones. I lost a teacher, mentor, confidant, and luminous presence in my life. I couldn't find the will to start a new therapeutic relationship, to retell my stories to a new stranger. I'd been there and done that. Maybe I could heal myself.

Us vs. Them

They like the word *team* in the workplace. Employers contrive ways to put individuals into teams because teamwork can increase efficiency, which remits financial benefits (for the employers). It's an imposed artifice, though in many of my old jobs it worked—there was a feeling of coming together to get the work done, of having each other's back, of being part of something bigger, even if it was just a group of young people getting a surge of customers fed to keep ourselves employed.

With this feeling of teamwork came a boost of positivity, and that could help you get through anything. But a team isn't born of a boss's declaration. A real team requires respect. The respect of your coworkers is essential in the ER, but it must be earned.

Everyone has a job to do according to their role, and each role is focused on the same mission—helping the patient. Teamwork should come easily, but competitiveness runs deep. The life-and-death stakes are just as likely to ramp up divisiveness as tamp it down. Perhaps this is true of any place full of highly competent people.

Newbies to the ER environment are warned that the staff is made up of people with "strong personalities." They need that strength to advocate for the patient, to insist the right thing is done the right way, to oppose a doctor when necessary. Doctors sometimes take on the entire medical system for a patient, drawing from a deep vein of stubborn will.

One challenge for me as a newbie was learning how to balance priorities I had for myself with the patients and the priorities nurses and doctors had for me. Advocates were often used to fetch—bring family members back to the room, carry messages to other staff, bring a patient a blanket, drink, or sandwich. Such tasks were fast and easy, but our work managing families during a code, assessing a possible child abuse case, or interviewing a victim of domestic violence had to be respected. It had to be OK to say "not now." Sometimes nurses would bristle when I insisted on following my hierarchy of tasks. Faced with an overwhelming workload, they were looking to delegate anything they could.

People driven toward lifesaving work often don't just *want* to make a difference—they *need* to make a difference. And some need their work to be recognized, not just on its own value, but as being better than their peers'. They want their helping excellence to bring attention to themselves. We call that a hero complex. Competitive attitudes can drive individuals toward higher competence, so sometimes this works in favor of the patient and can benefit the whole ER. But this attitude can also undermine the team.

The more your identity is wrapped up in your work, the more impact work-related issues have on your self-esteem and security. An ego under attack will launch all kinds of defenses to regain the comforting belief that it's the best. Hurt feelings are one of the most dangerous things that can happen to humans. We justify all sorts of bad behavior when we are wounded.

It's said that "nurses eat their young," because of the harsh treatment inexperienced nurses can get from the experienced ones. Every year some newbies quit because staff was mean to them or they didn't feel they got the support they needed to feel comfortable working in the ER.

Working in the ER is not for everyone. But as directors struggle to keep their ERs staffed, they work harder at getting the experienced workers to serve as mentors and supervisors for newbies rather than tossing those newbies into the deep end with no rope.

One director strove to build teamwork through recognition of our shared mission—our mutual need to make a difference. When it was

ER Appreciation Week, she had pins made that staff could attach to their badge tags. Each pin was in the shape of a starfish and inscribed with the words "I made a difference!"

A card was attached to the pin and told the story of a man who, upon finding starfish dying in the sand, went along the beach tossing them into the water. When someone questioned the logic of his actions—there were too many starfish to save them all, too many to make a difference—he tossed another one to safety and said, "Made a difference to that one!"

Ten years later, embracing a tough-guy bravado, staff would create a T-shirt for appreciation week: "Prepared for Everything, Surprised by Nothing." We had both warriors and caregivers in the ER, or maybe it's truer to say that we were all caregiver warriors.

$$\triangle$$

Our ER department, made up of almost a hundred total staff in those early days, was too big for the cushy feel of a close-knit team, but certain people regularly took certain shifts, and as they worked together over time, camaraderie and trust grew. You came to know who was capable of what, who you could ask for help, and who needed your help—even if they never asked.

Weekend shifts used to grow the strongest team, because the same nurses committed to the same two days. For a long time, my ER had Baylor shifts, named for Baylor University Medical Center, which had figured out the best way to get weekends covered consistently was to pay a higher wage to nurses who commit to work them.

On weekends there was a day shift, a night shift, and a few of us mid-shifters who straddled day and night. Working together each weekend, celebrating years of holidays and birthdays together, away from their families, these nurses turned into family. I was twenty-eight when I started working with them.

The weekend day-shifters needed their weekdays free usually to take care of children. They had other pursuits as well: farming, art, school, a new business, or even another nursing job during the week.

They brought in homemade foods and got together outside the ER for potluck parties and to do crafts. They were among the most experienced nurses in the department. They'd seen it all and weren't looking for excitement, yet the routine of other departments or medical offices didn't appeal to them. They were all older than me.

At seven p.m., the night-shifters arrived. Some had a set schedule of seven shifts on, seven shifts off, and would travel together on their week off. When they had shared meals, they brought out a grill (kept hidden from administration), which they set up on the ambulance dock after midnight. And if the ER emptied out in the wee hours of the morning, they circled up to play hacky sack. They were mostly single and all younger than me.

You didn't have to be a nurse to be on the Baylor team—plenty of other staff worked every weekend—but only nurses got Baylor pay. Weekends were my only shifts in the beginning, so the weekend team was the only one I could be a part of, yet I wasn't eligible for true membership. I didn't work every weekend; I worked every other, and my time was split from one in the afternoon to one in the morning, six hours on the day shift and six on the night shift.

I was usually too intimidated to go to the night-shifters' parties. Even before I was thirty, I felt old among them: I had two degrees, had married twice, and had two kids. I dreamed of traveling like they did, of a life balanced with challenging, well-paid work on one end and a freedom I'd never known on the other end. I envied them without truly wanting to be them—I knew better than to glamorize their work. I knew that I didn't have what it took to be a nurse, not by a long shot.

The few ER parties I did go to were awkward. If I brought my husband, he and the other spouses were relegated to spectator status, while ER staff sealed their bond with the only glue we had—our ER stories. Like working people everywhere, we defaulted to our narrow shared common experience. But we weren't making widgets. Our tales were saturated with melodrama, and telling them left a stain.

It reminded me of other teams, groups I'd been in, especially for theater or film production. A tremendous synergy is emitted as you create something together, but once you reach the end of the project, you experience a terrible deflation. You miss each other; you yearn to reexperience what you shared. But any attempt to do this is just an echo, a ghostly artifact of the real thing. Reminiscing could build an artificial bridge, but it didn't reach the emotions of the original experience or lead us anywhere new.

Gradually I increased the number of shifts I was assigned, taking weekday hours when my kids were in preschool. Once they were in middle school, I was promoted to manager. I had a tiny office, a former closet in the airlock—the space between the exterior doors of the ER and the doors opening to triage.

It was about a five-by-three-foot space. My desk was wedged in at one end with my chair. When someone entered, they had to stand up against the door. The door opened out to a row of registration desks. The window (there was a window!) opened to the airlock. I was inclined to leave the blinds open, on the chance that my daughter and her friend, out for a practice run with their school's cross-country team, would take a detour. They'd come and tap on my window, begging for candy. I was a welcome pit stop. But it was also mistaken for a cashier window—people would knock on the glass to ask directions or to try to pay their bill.

I can't recall how my office became the lactation room. As hard as it was to have time to sit and eat once in a twelve-hour period, getting away to pump breast milk was nearly impossible. We had few office spaces. A lactating mom could use the Family Room if it was empty, but it had no lock. I offered my office to one nursing mom, and she spread the word. I let the charge nurses know they could hand over the key whenever it was requested.

Pumping milk is a very private activity. An office in an airlock seems far from ideal, but the blinds could close, the door could lock, and no one was going to stumble in accidentally—it was a room hiding in plain sight. I had the inside painted eggplant purple and decorated it with quotes and images that inspired me. With tastes running to the woo-woo side of spiritual and politics left of center, I don't know what the nursing moms thought of the décor that surrounded them, but they surprised me by getting a bulletin board hung beside my desk—on the only wall big enough—and on it they tacked up a thank-you note from all of them with pictures of their babies.

I made some close friends in those years, opting for small pairings where we could link our ER life to our outside lives. These were the only people I could tell my uncensored ER stories; otherwise I kept the worst of them inside, not telling my husband or non-ER friends. I didn't want to spread secondary trauma around. I didn't want loving me to carry a penalty, an infection of nightmare images.

Yet I wanted to share. I wanted to lessen the horror and loneliness. I wanted those I loved to know something of my travels in this weird and frightening place, to understand how I was changing. But what if I was changing into someone they couldn't love? If I told them why I was changing, would they change as well? Perhaps my darkness was contagious, an uncurable virus. Not sharing my stories meant protecting my loved ones from all these painful vignettes and from the take-home message I was absorbing: The world is randomly terrifying.

If a patient died on one of my night shifts, I would sometimes come home late at night to a quiet house and light a candle. I'd sit still, watching it, trying to let go of the whirlwind of activity and emotions and send prayerful thoughts to the patient and family. I'd leave the candle there, and when I got up the next day my husband would make a gentle inquiry. But it felt wrong to burden him with the sadness, and I began to believe that if he didn't ask me, I could forget. I quit lighting candles. I just slipped into bed after my shift and closed my eyes, begging my mind to let go.

Writing shift reports gave me a way to process the surreal. When a director I was close to was reading my reports, I felt someone I trusted was tracking my journey. She read between the lines and checked in with me when she sensed a case was particularly hard. I took this lesson to heart and endeavored to do the same once I was a supervisor, leaving notes of support on the shift report, sending an email, or catching up with my teammates in person during their shift.

As the group of advocates grew, we turned to each other more. No one knew better the particular difficulties unique to our role, what we saw, heard, and dealt with. We became our own team. Everyone had a buddy or two they could trust with their spillover trauma, a partner willing to trade the saddest of sad stories.

But the advocate group wasn't immune from ER competitiveness. Among us also ran that undercurrent of scrutiny: *"I know I do this job better than you."*

△

When I worked in adoptions, I sometimes used an exercise from family psychotherapist Virginia Satir. She used a mobile to demonstrate how dynamics shift when a family member is added. This was useful with adoptive families who already had children older than preschool age.

I made a mobile with characters dangling down, a character for each family member. When I presented it to the family, I identified them as the characters and pointed out the balance, characters all dangling steadily, each in their place. "This is your family. Everyone has a place and there's balance. But when we add a new person . . ." I added a new element, an unknown character, and I pushed it into the center. All of the characters on the mobile went wonky, tipping to one side or the other. "It affects the entire family." The mobile was completely unbalanced.

I would adjust the characters' positions until it was once again stable, demonstrating that their family unit would again find its balance, but there would be this period of adjustment, and it might be unsettling. The family is a system, and changing its membership is a systemic change impacting each person.

When I made this mobile and tucked it into my briefcase, I was shy about bringing it out—it was homemade and hokey, but the kids seemed to like it. Their parents said they referred to it later, after placement, when family life became unsteady.

The ER team is fluid; dynamics change as the people change. Those strong personalities clash, but eventually the system adjusts as the people adjust, and equilibrium is achieved. Then new staff arrives, a new batch of strong personalities clashing with the old, and it goes topsy-turvy all over again.

△

My father, born into a poor Tennessee family, earned a place at West Point and climbed to the rank of colonel. He did not require me to address him or anyone else as "sir." I told myself that his fellow officers had to earn my respect. I didn't want to submit a "sir" automatically, but I found it was an easy gesture that made a conveniently positive impression. Under the cover of that deception, I could hide my ambivalence about the military.

I was proud of my father, and being part of an Air Force family was like belonging to a kind of team, but that didn't compensate for being the perpetual "new kid." No child has control over their parents' careers, but in our case, I knew that even my father was powerless to change our circumstances. His well-being relied on the temperament of whatever general he was serving. His life, our lives, depended on the politics of the commander in chief. When I was seven, he was sent to Vietnam. As his dependents, we got to choose where to live that year, but for all the other assignments we were transferred with him. There was no telling where we'd end up.

As an Air Force Brat, I was accustomed to a male-dominated structure and well aware of the pecking order. Teamwork is valued as long as it doesn't challenge the status quo of the hierarchy, much like in the ER. The fathers of my fellow Brats were mostly kind, gently funny, and emotionally contained. But I felt vulnerable to the unpredictable whims of the men in charge, who held our fates in their hands. A blade of fear ran just under the surface of my childhood. I couldn't openly fight it, so that fear was transmuted into resentment. Defiance was not an acceptable quality for anyone in the military, especially a child, a *girl* child, and especially in the South (where we were usually stationed).

I was in eighth grade when we were stationed in Warner Robins, Georgia. Dad got orders to transfer to Japan. My brother was a rising junior in high school, and I would be a freshman. The idea of moving to Japan was thrilling—finally somewhere exciting!—but the reality would be agonizing.

We had a dog, two cats, and a horse—they'd all be left behind. Also, Mom suffered with asthma and was told it might worsen from the air quality in Japan. Dad didn't like the job he would be assigned, so he played the only card he had. He couldn't refuse orders, so he retired.

For the first time in my life, I got to spend four years in one place. But that place was Montgomery, Alabama, where my mom's parents lived, and everyone seemed stuck in place—or maybe that's just high school everywhere. My dad got hired as an instructor at a local college. Once I graduated, I left town, finally able to make my own choice about where I wanted to live.

$$\triangle$$

As a young adult, I continued to bristle under any obligation to defer to someone purely because of his position instead of his character. *His*, because this came up almost exclusively with men. I'd chosen a profession dominated by women, but men still pulled most of the strings. At the adoption agency, my coworkers and supervisor were women, but the director was a man. It was the same at the psychiatric hospital where I did my internship, and at almost every job I'd had.

Doctors, mostly men, were part of the team. They probably thought they led the team, but it didn't seem that way to me. They were the undisputed boss of patient care, but women ran the ER. This was a surprise.

From what I read, saw, and experienced in hospitals, I expected to find doctors in charge. The doctors in my ER had become independent contractors shortly before I started in 1991. I was told this was happening in many ERs, a shift from the past, when physicians were hospital employees. They were still part of hospital committees, sought-after consultants about matters that impacted medical practice, but the logistics of running the department fell mostly to women: nurses, charge nurses, nurse managers, and the ER director. There were exceptions— men occasionally worked in all these roles, and there were a few female ER doctors. But each ER director I worked for was a woman.

I liked working with women; perhaps I preferred it. Most women want to fit in and feel connected. Being accepted means doing your share of the work and doing it well. These women were capable and confident and expected the same of me.

A few ER physicians still clung to the figurehead of authority when I arrived. I applied the same deference I learned in the Air Force. In place of the obligatory "sir," I said "doctor." I knew when to ask their permission and what they needed from me. I knew my place—the doctor was the boss of the patient, but not the boss of me.

When staff had a doctor-related issue, it was not usually with an ER doctor. Specialists or primary care physicians who came in to see a patient found the ER an awkward challenge, lashing out in frustration at times. They didn't know where we kept supplies, we didn't always have their preferred tools, they had to share nurses with other doctors and patients. They were outside the comfort zone of their offices, where everything was tailored to support their work. Here, they were just another health care professional doing a job, and they sometimes erupted in frustration, yelling for a nurse or shouting in anger when we couldn't produce the equipment they preferred. In contrast, ER docs knew that staff was juggling tasks and patients just as frantically as they were, doing their best to keep up with supplies and equipment, and that we had to work together to take care of everyone.

The doctor's dictation room was a tiny space within the large nurses' station. Both ER and non-ER docs sat there to document in charts. When the docs were ready to sit and dictate, if a chair wasn't there, they would have to pull one in. When a sign went up reading "Do not remove the tweed chairs from the dictation room," there was a reaction.

Fatigue fuels foolishness. Everyone was tired. When there was a chance to sit, everyone wanted a chair. Chairs did not stay where they were placed. They had wheels for a reason.

In a sea of blue-covered chairs, there were three chairs of a tweed-like fabric. These three became designated for the doctors, never to be used by staff. Mostly these chairs sat empty while nurses stood on their feet or sat on countertops.

Then one day, one of the tweed chairs went missing. A search was conducted—had it been rolled away to an office? No. To the registration area? No. The doctor who'd insisted on the sign was furious. The next day a picture was mysteriously tacked onto the break room bulletin board: "Tweed" had hit the road.

With a red kerchief on a stick slung over his back, Tweed was photographed rolling down the street away from the hospital, never to be seen again. Or so we thought. Pictures of Tweed making his way across the state found their way to the ER. Tweed hitching a ride in the back of a pickup truck, Tweed enjoying a moment by a water fountain in Savannah, Tweed fallen on hard times, wobbling down the railroad tracks. One time we thought he was coming home—a picture of Tweed in the OR! But he was just visiting cousins and soon went back on his way.

Years after the Tweed prankster moved away—a bighearted young man with a sparkle in his eye—I saw Tweed. He sat alone on a sidewalk behind the ER, just fifty yards from the ambulance dock. No one was in sight. He looked pensive, debating his next move. I was ambivalent. I wanted him back, yet I needed him to be free. I left him to decide his own fate and never saw him again, but his legend lived on. It was a story of playful subversion that delighted the staff and possibly embarrassed the doctors. No one got in trouble, and we all took ourselves and our petty divisions a little less seriously.

Every year new doctors were recruited, usually fresh out of residency. Their welcome to the ER was characteristic of their new home—dramatic. Once the new doc was oriented and no longer had an experienced colleague shadowing him, staff was watching—waiting for all the elements to align. The ER had to be just the right amount of busy, with no urgent patients on the doc's caseload, and the right staff (those willing to be naughty) in all the right positions.

It was a Sunday night, and there was a lull between ambulance arrivals. Patients in the lobby were waiting under an hour. No one had died or was actively dying, so no grieving family lined the hallway. The charge nurse was Marty, who was highly skilled, with a wicked sense of humor. When she came to me, she'd already coerced registration staff—she had a fake chart in hand. She recruited Gary, a nurse tech, to crawl into a body bag in the never-used shower where DOA (dead on arrival) patients were sometimes brought by EMS to be pronounced so they could go to the morgue or funeral home.

My job was to present the chart to Dr. Lowry, the new guy. I showed the chart to him and explained about shower pronouncements. He nodded and laid the chart under a stack; a deceased patient without family present was a low priority.

Marty got Susan, the unit secretary, to unzip Gary's body bag a little more and stay near him. Word spread among the staff that the game was afoot. Everyone kept doing their work, but with frequent glances toward the shower and Dr. Lowry. After a few minutes, I approached the doctor again, explaining that the funeral home wanted to transport the deceased. I said I needed the pronouncement so I could finish the necessary paperwork. Dr. Lowry sighed. He grabbed the clipboard. Susan darted in to zip the body bag up and dashed back out, just as Dr. Lowry and I arrived at the shower door. Behind our backs, Marty gestured to staff that the prank was about to go down.

The shower room was tiny, and when the heavy door shut behind us, Marty, Dr. Lowry, and I were pressed tight against the gurney— nowhere to run. Outside the door stood a few nurses and techs, the unit secretaries watching from the nursing station and the ambulance crew peeking out their window, all in gleeful anticipation.

Inside the shower room, I was at the foot of the gurney to avoid being struck by a body flailing in panic. Dr. Lowry began to unzip the body bag. Gary had his eyes closed. Once the bag was opened to his chest, Gary's eyes flew open, and he yelled "HA!" Dr. Lowry jumped, his hands out to keep the gurney away. He spun to the door, and as he wrestled with the latch, the laughter around him finally registered. Gary sat up, howling, the body bag limp around him. Marty seemed more contained but had a wide grin and took her glasses off to wipe away a tear. I chuckled in relief, worried that the prank would go sideways, always feeling sorry for the new doc and the deceitful role I played.

The shower door opened from the outside and staff peeked in, eager to see the aftermath, wide-eyed as children on Christmas morning. The story was told to our coworkers, over and over, until everyone that played a part in it no longer worked in the ER. It was wrong in all sorts of ways, but the doctors were good sports. The ability to bear a humiliating prank with humor was key to their joining our team. One time a new doctor told me he knew he was being set up for a prank but went along anyway. He knew the importance of initiation.

Once they were part of us, many doctors seemed to find leaving the ER as hard as I did. But some realized early on that it wasn't for them, eventually not only leaving our ER but the practice of ER medicine altogether. One doctor left to create a free clinic for our community, one we could refer indigent patients to. Another doctor left to work at an urgent care clinic. He left the staff a gift, a picnic table that sat on a tiny square of grass by the ambulance dock. Until that space was overtaken by an expansion of the ER, it was a place we could sit to briefly feel the sun we otherwise didn't see during our long shifts. Another doctor joined the hospital's IT department, to improve the physician computer interface, and one became part of the medical school's administration.

Each year there was a trickle of new doctors coming in and one or two leaving. Most of the new doctors didn't want to climb onto the authoritarian platform of the past. Some bold ones made this clear on day one: "Call me Steve." I didn't call him "Steve," not at first, trusting my experience with authority more than I trusted "Steve." But, as time and trials proved Steve to be reasonably easy to work with, I might use his first name, especially in the break room or outside the ER—but only as a careful choice, never as a casual habit. There was a power differential between doctors and everyone else, and that blade of fear from my childhood told me to never forget it.

My ability to display deference (often insincere) came from being around officers in the military. I credit those childhood experiences for my savvy with physicians, my lack of run-ins—though one did ask me out on a date, knowing I was married, and another used his brute strength to mark territory.

He was a surgeon, not one of "our" docs. I met him as I walked a family to the surgery waiting room. A burly man known for his temper. I courteously introduced him to the family. He turned to me: "And you are?"

"Kathryn Kyker, a social worker from the ER. I've been working with the Jennings family since their son came in."

"Nice to meet you." He gave a small smile and offered his hand. It was unusual for a doctor to be so formal to staff. He enveloped my hand in his claw, where he proceeded to crush it. I winced, but he didn't let go. I knew what this was—a childish show of strength by someone in a high position riddled with insecurity. I held on with a steely expression until he let go. I said my goodbyes to the family, walked down the corridor, and waited till I was out of sight to cradle my throbbing hand. I was the queen of strong handshakes and despised a limp one— this had never happened. I wish I'd called him out, even making a joke of it, right in the moment, forcing an insincere apology out of him. Enduring the pain without complaint made me feel strong, but I was the only one hurt from that interaction—I played right into his hand.

This team of my early years, the "old ER," fell apart as a new ER was constructed. A chasm grew between the changes my first ER director thought were best for patients and staff and what the doctors felt they needed. Among the areas of conflict were disputes about a new triage system, and how we would manage flow during the construction phase. Our director won those battles but paid the price when top administration supported the doctors' call for a change in leadership. The new ER featured the changes she'd fought for, but she wasn't there to see it. Almost half of the ER staff left in the months following her departure. She had hired me. My position existed because of her vision; she created my career.

I wanted to show her my appreciation, my loyalty, to join my friends who left in protest in a show of support, and I wanted to keep working with her, but my beloved boss was a victim of her own success. Our role was unique; I wouldn't find a comparable position in another ER. And, thanks to her, I had a group of advocates to supervise. Leaving them amid such workplace turmoil felt unthinkable. My loyalty came up against a sense of commitment to the advocates, my family, and even myself—I had worked hard to get the position I had. I resolved my ambivalence about staying by making work only about work, certain I could separate my ER life from my non-ER life. I would not get personally invested. I would just do the job for as long as I had to.

I joined Facebook, but I didn't friend any ER staff. My team was gone.

Those that remained after the mass exodus retreated to their respective corners. This was simplified by two things the doctors lobbied for in the new ER—a separate break room that stayed locked, and their own work area outside of the nurses' station (with chairs that stayed in place). Being in their own space near each other would enhance *their* teamwork, they said, but diminished the feeling of their being part of our team. No longer sharing a workspace decreased our communication, both professional and personal. Our paths only overlapped in patient rooms, unless one of us sought out the other.

The smallest change may have been the most telling—new doctors were no longer initiated by the staff. Our ritual prank, staging a death to scare the new doc, no longer made sense. They were no longer joining our team.

There were many doctors I continued to enjoy working with, and we chatted amicably in and outside of the ER. They were conscientious and kind and supported my efforts. They bought the staff pizza when we were slammed and sent me flowers when my father died. I saw them engage compassionately with difficult patients, comfort frightened children, go out on a limb with colleagues when a patient couldn't afford follow-up care, and take on administrators when a patient needed tests or admission but didn't fit the criteria. I was grateful when ER doctors took care of my husband's hand injury, my mother-in-law's ministrokes, and my mother's heart palpitations.

When I crashed on a bike trail, I sheepishly asked one to check out my hematoma, which was the size of a large potato bulging below my navel. She graciously gave me a quick and private assessment, which kept me from having to check in and be subjected to tests I didn't need, avoiding the subsequent large bill and saving me the embarrassment of exposing my middle-aged tummy to my other coworkers.

I could have called many doctors by their first names to chip away at some of the formality dividing us, but I never did that again. The power differential was real, and this was one way to remember it.

△

The few ER friendships that sustained me the last half of my career that continue now are those rich enough to block the glare of our time on the ER stage so that we can move beyond it. I didn't look for friends who resonated with the ER drama but for those who were interested in the world beyond it. Best of all, my friends make me laugh.

Finding few friends in a place full of coworkers was not a new situation for me. I grew up being the outsider, seeking soulmates, and, in their absence, settling for acquaintances that were at least diverting. Among the two dozen people working an ER shift, there were always a few I could count on for anything.

In the first years, my shifts were usually twelve hours long. When I arrived, I checked the whiteboard where the names of nurses were written by their areas of assignment, and I plotted my day. I noted my go-to nurses in each area for questions, assistance, or empathy if I needed to vent about a difficult patient, family, or doctor.

"How long are you in for?" I'd ask my coworkers when I didn't know their schedule. They laughed at the prison comparison, but sometimes, to us non-convicts, a shift felt like doing time. When the day was dragging, I knew where to go to make the clock run, who would give me gardening tips, recommend books, talk films with me, or tell me stories. Visiting a favorite nurse at triage was the best option back in the day when there were pauses between the flow of patients, or, when it was busy, helping the nurse manage the flow—getting the sickest to the front of the line.

I'd also peek in the window to see who was working dispatch for the ambulance crew. They were based in the ER back then and would hang out between calls, often helping the nurses work a trauma. I depended on them for a heads-up on risks and complications associated with an incoming patient's home environment and relationships.

Even on the busiest day, a twelve-hour stretch afforded moments to slow down, and I wanted to spend those slower moments with good company. I learned to pace myself to reserve some energy for the final hours of my shift.

The last advocate scheduled at night couldn't leave until every assessment and intervention was wrapped up. Those shifts could go much longer than twelve hours, exceeding that reserve of energy, consuming the precious hours when you should be sleeping before coming back to do it all again. A solid coworker could ease this relentless tedium.

By the time we were in the newly built ER, the number of patients waiting to be seen was rapidly climbing, while staffing levels for the advocates remained the same. I worked faster and faster just to keep up. Slow times became rare. When they did happen, I no longer indulged in chats at the nurses' station. Instead, I dove into a never-ending list of management projects, thinking I could get it all done if I never stopped doing.

Once the increase in patients lasted long enough to prove it wasn't a temporary surge, the hiring increased, especially of nurses and techs. Soon most of the staff was much younger than me. I didn't get to know them, didn't discover what shared interests we had that might divert us from a tedious shift and connect us during a painful one.

Then, in a cost-saving move that took us by surprise, the ambulance crew was disbanded. A private company was hired, which wasn't based in our ER. This was happening in other hospitals, but we never thought it would happen to us. The medics' space was gobbled up by other hospital services. We saw our old paramedic friends only briefly, when they brought us patients as employees with the new company. This was one of many painful changes from the familiar old ways, made in hopes of sustaining the hospital's growth. We could no longer go to dispatch with questions about the scene when the patient couldn't respond; medics weren't in the department to give an extra hand when nursing was overwhelmed by trauma patients. We lost our friends, and the medics lost resources. They couldn't ask an advocate the best homecare options for a patient who wouldn't come in, and our doctors and nurses weren't easily accessible to explain new equipment and processes. We were now just another hospital to them instead of *their* hospital. Another blow to the former strength of our team.

When I went months without seeing a favorite medic from the early days, I put the word out to staff. I had no idea if he had moved to a different service, retired, or gotten hurt—as paramedics often do. He was already a grizzled, experienced medic when I was brand new. But with a quick smile, he was kinder to newbies than most of the paramedics—in fact, he supervised me for a "ride along" as part of my orientation. Joining him and his partner on one of my first mornings in the ER, I recall feeling nauseous sitting in the back of the ambulance, as he cared for an elderly lady we transported. Besides a fear of throwing up, I was, of course, worried about fainting, but his gentle spirit was comforting to me and the patients. Whenever he was on duty, he was my go-to paramedic for information, the one who wouldn't snarl at me for asking a stupid question and would help in any way he could.

Eventually my inquiries reached him, and he came to find me after transporting a patient. He remarked that he often spotted me in the ER, but I was "always so busy." He didn't want to interrupt me even to say hi.

"She was so busy" seemed likely to be my epitaph.

Now in retirement, there are times when I miss the feeling of being part of something big, of having a clear role that locks seamlessly into place with others and contributes to a shared goal of healing. But those feelings were strongest when we were inside someone's nightmare scenario made real. We were at our best when someone else was in profound pain and jeopardy.

I cannot call up the good without recalling the bad. But I can separate the team itself from the team*work*. I cherish my memories of coworkers, the ones I started with, the ones I ended with, and all those in between. They worked hard, they cared deeply, and when I let them, they eased me through shift after shift.

The Dark Side of Hope

The charge nurse worked to keep the fear out of her voice as she told me what was coming to trauma room one. She was being careful with me. My adrenaline surged. "We're getting three patients from a car accident, twin infants and their mom. We think they're OK, but there was a fatality on the scene, in their car." The fatality was an adult male, probably the woman's husband and the children's father.

When I walked into the room, the babies, two boys about a year old, were already in the arms of nurses. A paramedic guided the mom into the room and then went to whisper her report to the nurse.

The mother stood alone, crying, her stringy hair brushing her young shoulders, where red abrasions from a seat belt were visible around the straps of her camisole. The staff eyed the mom warily. If she had been on a gurney, they would have jumped into action, into their well-practiced routines, but in the absence of a clear medical issue, they hung back. Experience has taught us it's wise to give emotional trauma some physical space. Grief is a shape-shifting animal. We stand back to see if it's going to lash out at us.

But it was my job to move forward. I went to the mom's side. I told her who I was and that I would help her. I may have said that I was sorry for what happened, leaning on safe words open to her interpretation, purposefully vague, unsure how much she knew, how much she would let herself know. Her constant flood of tears indicated that she knew her husband was dead.

I could imagine the chaos at the wreck: children crying, medics scurrying around to get everyone except him loaded for the ER. The absence of activity around his body could tell her everything.

Before the medics arrived, she was in the car beside him. Maybe he talked to her, but most likely he was not responsive at all. Maybe she talked to *him*. It comforts me to believe that. I imagine myself in that car, talking to him, even if I didn't know him. Survivors of car crashes seem to know when there's a fatality in the car, even with the distraction of their own injuries.

Medical care comes before conversation. Once patients are cleared of significant injuries, they will be told if someone died in the accident. Usually their family tells them, sometimes the police, but we don't leave that to chance. We know the impact death can have, the range of shocked reactions. Upon hearing the news, if they have chest pain or elevated blood pressure, or they fall out, we know how to respond. We also know the power of denial, the seductive way it blocks the truth, for good or ill.

Elsewhere in medicine, hope is revered as an essential ingredient in healing, but in the ER, we are stingy with hope. We have seen its dark side. We manage the dose, doling it out in tentative measures. In the absence of our frank notification of death, people will cling to a sliver of hope and build it into a full-fledged belief. They are trying to keep from being unmoored, but we cannot allow it.

We are responsible for helping them take steps toward their new reality. We can't fix that wound, but in the acute stage of grief the ER can function like a padded cell—no real comfort but basic safety—able to absorb implosions and explosions.

If they are hurt badly enough to need admission, we delay telling them about the death unless they ask. We know that emotional pain can wipe out your strength, compromise your ability to heal physically.

We work with the family who comes to visit our patient. Before bringing them to the room, we explain what we know and what the patient may not know. Families make their own choice about the telling. We think it's better for the patient to hear bad news from their family, from someone intimately connected to them. Understandably, families can be as reluctant as we are to impart those heartbreaking details.

One time a family member told me that she didn't want to be the one remembered as telling a family member about a death. She said it like it would be a mark against her, a permanent dark shadow on the relationship. I had never thought about it like that. If a stranger tells you that your loved one has died, does the memory of that stranger persist—the one who upended your reality? If so, I am stuck in the traumatic memories of so many people. I pray that my image is soft around the edges, that they know I cared, that they and their loved one mattered to me.

There was no family to tell this patient that her husband died, and she didn't ask. Still standing upright in the trauma room, she suddenly wailed that it was her fault, that she loved him, and that it should have been her. We eased her onto a stretcher and into a gown. I told her he wouldn't want it to be her, that it was an accident. She shook her head, not accepting comfort from a stranger who knew nothing of her life with the man she'd lost.

The doctor moved from assessing the children to the mom. She had a sore shoulder from the seat belt and a sore leg. She would need X-rays. I asked who she wanted me to call to be with her and help with the kids. Her mother lived many states away. Her father lived closer, but she never talked to him and didn't have his number. She said she had no friends. "I only had him; he was my life."

Now I was scared. I had a grieving widow with possible injuries, who had two babies and no one to call. But almost no one really has *no one*. Sometimes the connections they have are just too frayed to risk reaching out. My job was to find the leads they didn't want to give, probing those frayed connections. She let me call her boss.

She had just taken a job at a fast-food place; her boss was a man who sounded very kind on the phone. I told him what happened, even about the fatality. Did she have any coworkers that would help? He said he would help. I told him they were living in a hotel with payment due. They needed their room paid for so they could return there, so their stuff wouldn't be tossed out. He said he would pay the bill.

I went back to the room. A nurse and a tech held the children, who were uninjured. Mom was back from X-ray. She asked for her husband—where was he, was he brought here, how was he? The staff and I exchanged "uh-oh" looks. We thought her earlier words and tears meant she knew, but none of us had spoken the truth plainly. I told the patient I would find out. I went to the doctor. He would come and play his part: official bearer of the worst news.

Once it's clear that notification of a death must be done, it seems cruel to delay. I have done the telling many times, and I believe I do it as well or better than most physicians, in terms of connecting to the bereaved and being straightforward but kind. But I cannot inhabit the archetypal presence that a doctor provides, and I've come to recognize the importance of such a role during these times.

Whether it's due to our own experience, stories from our family, or all those medical dramas, we expect to hear about matters of life and death from The Doctor. And having those expectations met helps in some tiny way, like being part of a ritual we didn't know we wanted or needed. Giving a nod to this need is the least we can do in the ER. For some, a doctor taking the time to talk to them about the death is a sign of respect for their loss—the man or woman in a white coat showed up to deliver the news. It's a larger-than-life moment and calls for a larger-than-life person. Thankfully most doctors know the importance of playing this part, even when they did not personally provide care to the patient. But the man or woman in the white coat also knows that grief can go sideways, so they take us with them. They need only to say the words and they can leave. But we stay.

The doctor told the patient—the wife who survived the car accident, the mother with two babies—that her husband died in the crash. She wanted to deny it, but her protests lacked conviction. She cycled through her mantra of it being her fault, it should have been her, and what would she do without him? Then she asked for her mother.

I was surprised to hear that she spoke with her mother in the ambulance, even as her conversation interfered with the efforts of the medics. For patients who remain conscious, the cell phone can be an impediment on the scene, as patients insist on making a call, often still talking as they roll into the ER. Some doctors tell them to get off the phone, others walk out of the room, telling the staff to come get them when the patient's ready.

All of us want to reach out and touch someone familiar when we feel alone at a scary time. These conversations feel like lifelines. But delaying the start of an IV or the positioning of a neck collar can have dire consequences.

For this patient, now was time to get on the phone. She told her mother the news. The patient got quiet, listening. It became apparent that the mother was not saying words of comfort. The patient's face contorted with pain, and she moaned in an anguished protest, "Mom!" She handed me the phone. On the other end, her mom handed her phone to a friend.

The friend said to me, "We want to know what really happened. She's known to exaggerate."

"I heard what she told you, and it was correct. She and her family were in a car crash, and her husband died on the scene. She and the kids are OK, but they need support."

The friend relayed this to the mom. "Well," the friend said with authority, "you have to keep her to make sure she gets the help she needs."

"There's no medical reason for admission. She's going to be discharged, and I hope she won't be alone with the kids."

"You need to find her help, someone to take care of the kids."

I thought, somewhat sarcastically, that it must be lovely to believe our world is like that, where such help exists and can be activated by my making a phone call. After all, we do have shelters for the unhoused and victims of domestic abuse, foster care for children, psychiatric facilities for those with mental health crises (all of these difficult to get in), but immediate care for a grieving woman on the edge with two young children—that's where family steps in. If you don't have family, or they aren't willing and able, then maybe close friends, or a church. No hardship fairies await a summons from my wand.

There were organizations that might help her at some point, but no one to pick her up from the ER and stay by her side through the next days. Her mother would not be coming.

I've learned from talking to parents who choose not to step in that such refusals are often shaped by a history—bridges were torched, painfully rebuilt, only to be torched again. When you hear the whole story, it becomes much harder to judge. I could imagine myself in their shoes, agonizing over how much the past should influence the present.

Some parents have simply run out of help to give and are depleted financially and emotionally. Trying to help now may cost them their own health. Refusing my request might mean they are finally protecting themselves, and often they confess this to me in tones full of shame and grief. Though I need them, I don't exploit their guilt. But I do paint the picture in all its matter-of-fact bleakness.

The picture painted itself in this situation: her daughter's husband was dead, her daughter was on the edge of homelessness in addition to being in the throes of acute grief, with two very young children dependent on her. If this picture didn't move the mom to act, what would? I had invested all my hope in that mom. I hung up the phone knowing that the dark place I sat in with the patient just got darker.

The edges of this case blur into others. I think that the kind employer and his wife came to pick her up and took her to the hotel, that he told me he had food for her and the children. I gave him the ER number, in case he had questions about resources we gave her, in case he got stuck and needed our help. He told me that he and his family would take care of them.

I want to remember it this way. But my imagination may be filling in the blanks, spinning an ending that allows me to sleep.

It's hard to explain how someone in such a perilous situation does not qualify for admission. Well, it's easy to explain—she didn't have a medical need for admission. It's hard to *justify*. There are so many needs that go beyond what a hospital is set up to do, so many ways that people fall through our threadbare safety nets. Often our only choice is to return you to the place you came from, even if it's not perfect—our feeble Band-Aid drooping over too big a wound.

There was someone, one person, committed to checking on her, to helping her, and that one person was not related to her, hardly knew her at all. In fact, he was from another country. I wondered what he thought of her isolation, how alienated she was from her family and resources. I wondered if he was surprised that he was the only one we found willing to help her, and whether people took better care of each other in his country of birth.

They Can't Take This Away from Me . . . Can They?

In my early years, as I worried about my coworkers discovering my aversion to blood and the taunting sure to follow, I found comfort in the discovery of a fear most of them shared that was seemingly more ridiculous than any of my fears: They were terrified of babies! Some were intimidated by the high-stakes conversions necessary to adapt lifesaving measures to a tiny human, and some had a generalized "I don't do kids" aversion. But nearly every ER nurse's ultimate nightmare scenario was caring for a mom in labor.

Because this fear was common among ER staff, it wasn't a secret they kept from each other, just from the world at large, especially the pregnant moms and their family members. But I was delighted by this discovery and didn't try to hide it.

There were few instances when I could feel courageous in comparison to my coworkers. Unlike most nurses, I had a high tolerance for staying in emotional chaos, being present when there was nothing to do, no way to make it better. I could sit with that, knowing that the only thing worse than being there would be to abandon the person already isolated by their pain.

Nurses cannot stand being helpless. They throw themselves into tangible tasks. They put their skills and knowledge on the line every day, patient after patient. And though they build on that foundation, their routines change with the science. The hospital continually adopts new equipment, protocols, and medications requiring complex delivery. ER nurses are constantly receiving training. Their motto is "Watch one, do one, teach one." They can apply something they learned months ago to today's real-time crises. A willingness to learn, to rise to such challenges, is essential for ER nurses, but confidence comes with practice and feeling prepared. That's one reason why a newborn strikes such deep terror. ER staff exude a confidence that comes off as cockiness, but newborns render them helpless and humble.

Moms in labor get diverted to the maternity unit. Nurses become track stars when confronted with a woman having strong, rapid contractions. A shout of "Tell L&D we're coming!" emits from a blur of a nurse hurtling down a hallway with a woman in a wheelchair. Sometimes they don't make it—the woman delivers in the elevator. A nurse's speed can make the difference between not having to handle the birth at all and having to handle it completely—and all alone.

If the dad is parking the car, he's left out altogether. The nurse is in a race against contractions to get the laboring woman up to the unit where they are not afraid of babies. Because births happen so rarely in the ER, an ER nurse never feels prepared for a baby, even if she's had one.

This amused me to no end. It was one of the many ways that I was so fundamentally different from my coworkers. I'd had two children, and while I might share that I'd had "natural births," I didn't share that I'd birthed my children at home. I assumed that I would be mocked for this. This choice of mine was controversial back when I chose it. My family, acquaintances, and even total strangers expressed concerns and criticisms, as pregnancy seems to give others a free pass to overstep social boundaries.

Working in the world of medicine, I realized that my home births would be perceived not only as foolhardy but also as a rejection of almighty Medicine. I was embedded in a community of believers, trying to keep my skeptic status undercover.

Other countries treat birth as a normal process usually needing little medical intervention. I am grateful that my friends who needed C-sections or had other birthing emergencies got the care they needed, and I shudder at the thought of that care not being immediately available for everyone. But a medical approach can complicate the birth process; monitoring and medications can prompt more medical interventions, as they slow down or complicate the natural process. I'm not advocating for reducing any medical options, but I'd also like to see more options for noncomplicated deliveries.

When confronted by a birth in progress, the ER—land of worst-case scenarios—assumes there will be a medical complication. Equipment rarely seen must be found. Staff huddle around it, whispering urgent reminders about its use. If there are specific OB rooms (with exam tables with stirrups), the patient may be placed in one, but often these patients—women having babies—are put in the most tricked-out trauma room because that's where the lifesaving equipment is: masks, tubing for airway protection, and the code cart full of medications.

Time spent setting a room up for a birth is better spent getting the woman to the OB floor. But if a woman is pushing or the baby's head is already crowning, the ER accepts their fate: This is their patient, and where there is now one, there will soon be two. When there is no time to get the patient upstairs, we do the next-best thing and call Labor and Delivery nurses to come to the ER.

Usually arriving just after delivery, the L&D nurses, accustomed to the tiniest patients, sweep in and whisk the baby into arms to assess and treat as needed. They must love this shift in power, stealing the treasure, the glory, our hero's cape right off us, but I never noticed them gloating—I was too busy.

I learned that I had a place in these trauma rooms. While everyone else was focused on the lower half of the gurney, I stationed myself at the head of the bed, where there was plenty of room because no one stood there, to talk to the mom, hold her hand, or breathe through the contractions with her. Staff was at the foot of the bed, ready to save her life and the life of her child.

If the patient came by ambulance, in the moments before arrival I would sometimes hear a nurse or tech repeat what the medics had said on the radio, whether the mom had a health condition, whether she had an obstetrician. Often, she had no physician and no prenatal care. Under the spell of fear that the ER concocts, staff would whisper, "No ultrasound, no prenatal care. There's no telling what's going to come out." I would lean in and gleefully tell them that I knew exactly what was going to come out—a baby!

Here was something I remembered about the real world, something I cherished and clung to. I held it up to shine some light on the creeping shadows.

In that real, before-the-ER world, I wasn't prepared to be pregnant. I didn't have a doctor, or insurance, or any familiarity with babies. I was a grad student, twenty-three, recently divorced, and in a new relationship. I was overwhelmed by the idea of parenting, but I loved my baby. I wanted him no matter what. I didn't have to get married. I intended to say no if offered a proposal, or at least, "Let's wait." But inexplicably, I heard myself say yes, and I married the baby's father the next month in his brother's backyard with friends and family, me in a wedding dress made by my best friend. Despite this dubious start, I was hopeful. My husband was not afraid of babies.

Having denied my way through the first trimester, I quickly looked for care. I could not find an OB in town that would take me as a patient without insurance or a large down payment on the enormous costs to come. An acquaintance who was a nurse (but not in the ER) told me about a local midwife practice. There were lay midwives in our town who attended home births, but this was a practice of two certified nurse midwives. To provide me with pre- and postnatal care and attend home births, they had to comply with state laws and the requirements of their profession and have physician backup.

No physician in our town would back them up, but they had found a supportive physician group in a nearby town. I visited that practice twice for those doctors to examine me and order tests as needed. They consulted with the midwives about my progress or any concerns. If I needed to deliver in a hospital, I would go to their rural hospital about forty minutes away. But if there was an emergency, I'd go to my town's ER, the one less than a mile away, the one that would become my work home a few years later.

The midwives explained what would happen if I went to the ER: "They probably won't let us in your room. They don't like what we do, and they may not be nice to you. They may scold you for trying to have a baby at home . . . *but they will take care of you.*"

I didn't have to go to the ER. I had a healthy baby boy at home with my midwives, my husband, and my best friend at my side.

When I was close to developing a breast infection, the midwives increased their postnatal visits and helped me recover. When the love I felt for my son leapt over every emotional boundary I ever constructed and overwhelmed my heart, they watched me for postpartum depression and kept visiting me. No friends of mine had babies yet; I was out of sync with my generation. They gave me information on a local support group, and I met other new moms.

When I got pregnant again, I became the first repeat customer for this team of midwives. I had another healthy baby at home, this time a girl. When she had mild jaundice, the midwives' attention kept her out of the hospital. I cannot imagine myself or my children getting better care.

A planned home birth comes with homework. In my first meeting with the midwives, they asked about my motivation. I cited the financial issues. They told me that worries about costs would not get me through labor. If money was my primary motivation, I would most likely end up in the hospital when the pain and fear hit hard. I set about changing my motivation.

I read about the differences between giving birth in the United States and everywhere else, how we medicalize the process and yet still have poor statistics in comparison to countries with comparable medical technology.[1] I read labor stories written by women giving birth or in attendance. Those stories were not perfect; things sometimes went wrong. But since I was a healthy young woman, my child and I were at low risk. Still, my husband and friend had to learn infant CPR, and the midwives' bag included oxygen, a scalpel, and sutures.

---

1. "Women in the U.S. More Likely to Die in Pregnancy, Childbirth, and Postpartum Than Women in Other High-Income Nations," The Commonwealth Fund, released November 18, 2020, https://www.commonwealthfund.org/press-release /2020/women-us-more-likely-die-pregnancy-childbirth-and-postpartum-women -other-high.

I bought absorbent pads to go under me and over my mattress. We found a bucket for the placenta.

Home births are not for everyone, but I feel profoundly lucky that in the late eighties, this option with certified nurse midwives was available in my community. In the nineties, due to pressure from local physicians, that option disappeared from my town and has not returned. But it could be even worse—I do not live in a "maternity care desert."[2]

The March of Dimes' report on the worsening state of maternal health (released September 2024) provides data showing no or limited maternity care services in more than one-third of US counties, disproportionately affecting women of color and low-income women. But in non-rural areas, births can be a moneymaker. Long ago, hospitals changed their rules and processes and made birthing rooms homey. Women now have a better chance of directing their birthing experience, but that experience will usually be within the confines of the medical industry, if you're lucky enough to live in an area with obstetric resources at all.

Although my birthing experience could not be more different, I could relate to the women who gave birth in our ER. I knew how scary it was to be pregnant and poor. I could understand not getting prenatal care. I knew denial. I could relate to having to come to the ER to give birth because that could have happened to me.

Those I worked beside revered the world of medicine—the antidote to their own "what if" fears. The power of their belief wormed its way into my mind and body. The births I was present for in the ER were normal deliveries with healthy babies. But we also saw many pediatric injuries, infant deaths, and miscarriages. If I had gotten pregnant after I started working in the ER, I don't think I would have considered a home birth. I would have been too frightened by the worst-case scenarios. Anything could happen—who knew what may come out?

I cherish my birthing memories, that I brought my children into the world in my own home with four people present—all of whom I loved and trusted with my life and the life of my child. That birthing

2. "Nowhere to Go: Maternity Care Deserts Across the US," March of Dimes, accessed 2024, at https://marchofdimes.org/maternity-care-deserts-report.

team stayed with me twelve, sixteen, perhaps twenty hours straight. They didn't change shift; there wasn't a new nurse coming on, a doctor going off call, or a need for my labor and the baby's birth to adhere to a schedule.

There was also no one to clean up. The placenta sat in the bucket in our bathtub until my husband buried it in the garden.

It was the perfect mess that is real life. The beauty of those experiences stands untouched by the ER's grasp of cold dread. I'm glad for who I was then, *how* I was then—sorting out my new life as best I could, able to imagine that everything was going to be just fine.

ACT

How to Have
a Good* ER Visit

1. **Manage your expectations.**
   Cures are improbable, and significant insights into chronic ailments are unlikely.
2. **Come early if you want to leave on the same day.**
   Allow eight hours for your visit, and more if we're busy. (Will it really take eight hours?! See #1.)
3. **Prepare to tell us your name and date of birth at least ten times.**
   After the first five times, patients get frustrated, thinking we are not listening, not writing it down, or not reading the chart. But we're required to take this safety step to ensure you are you, each time we take something from you, put something in you, expose you to radiation, or penetrate your skin with pointy implements.
4. **Your chart doesn't tell us everything we need to know.**
   Patients dismiss questions about their medical history with "It's in my chart." The chart could be wrong or unclear. Sometimes the chart is not immediately accessible. Sometimes we just want to hear it in your words.
5. **Bring someone with you.**
   When you finally go to the bathroom in the waiting room, that's when we'll call your name. Someone needs

* "Good" being relative to how bad a bad experience can be.

to stay and listen for your name, convince staff that you're still here, and run to get you before the nurse skips to the next name.

6. **That someone needs to be sober.**
   The person with you needs to be able to drive you home so that you're able to receive pain medication if necessary. That person also needs to be a helpful sort, someone who makes things better.

7. **Know your primary complaint.**
   When the nurse asks why you're here, don't start with "Ten years ago . . ." Start with what's happening today and work your way back. Focus on your main problem.

8. **Do not lie.**
   About your drug use, about your phone number, or about your symptoms. If you try to jump the line by feigning worse symptoms, you will be found out and despised for endangering a sicker patient.

9. **Don't rate your pain as an "eleven" on the one-to-ten pain scale.**
   Elevens reek of attention-seeking. Be honest. Rating your pain as a ten means it's the worst pain you've ever felt. Is it? Truly?

10. **Have your helpful person wipe off the bed rails and anything else you expect to touch.**
    Should staff do this before you get in the room? Yes. Did they do it . . . ?

11. **Do not choose internet search results over the opinion of the trained professional evaluating you.** Ask the doctor for clarification, get a second opinion if needed, but don't assume that AI or your google skills are equal to their expertise.

12. **Put your phone down each time the doctor or staff enters your room.**
    It's in your best interest to give them your full attention.

13. **Don't rush out.**

    Check your discharge paperwork before you leave the room. Make sure that your name is on it. It should include your diagnosis, details of the recommended next steps (follow-up), and what you should do at home to ease your symptoms. The nurse should review this with you. Imagine yourself at home and consider the questions that may arise. Ask those questions now. If the nurse doesn't have the answer, ask them to check with the doctor. Wait in the room or just outside of it. Once you're out of the ER, you're no longer their patient. Calling back is problematic. Your providers may be gone or busy caring for the patient in front of them.

14. **Wash your hands as you exit.**

    When you get home, take a shower, and throw your clothes in the washer.

15. **The next day, when you wake up with the same complaint, see tip #1.**

The Devil You Know

My first ten years in the ER I worked part-time so that I could continue working with adoptive families for the private adoption agency. Once my kids were both in school, I added a few short weekday ER shifts in addition to my long shifts every other weekend.

Our team of advocates grew from three to eight, and our hours expanded from covering the ER ten hours a day to eighteen hours a day. This increase in our coverage was in response to the growing patient census. When I started, we saw about a hundred patients a day. Ten years later, the average was one hundred twenty patients a day. Twenty patients more a day adds up to about six hundred more a month, over seven thousand more in a year.

We no longer depended on other hospital departments for social service interventions that we could manage. We took call, so if an advocate wasn't in the ER when needed, the charge nurse called us in. We began to influence policies about the ER's response to reporting abuse, neglect, and assault. We strengthened our knowledge of community resources. Acknowledging our value and envisioning our potential, the ER director created a new position to strengthen the advocate role—an ER case manager who would provide supervision of the advocates as well as follow up with patients.

△

I enjoyed my work with adoptive families, but as a contract worker, I didn't receive benefits from that agency. I didn't get the warm feeling of belonging to a team that worked together in the trenches. I worked alone with my caseload of adoptive parents, and at the end of each meeting, they handed me a check, a portion of the total cost for their home study. It went straight to the agency but gave a transactional feel to the work.

Each case was a family with a slightly different version of the same story: When I met them, they wanted a child, and when I left them, they had a child. Each story had its own twists and turns, and each placement was immensely satisfying, but each time I started and stopped in the same place. I was ready for more.

Most of the adoptions were international—US couples adopting children from other countries. I wanted to believe that I was part of making a difference to a child in need, but we couldn't know the true circumstances of why the child was available for adoption. There was no way to know the ethics of countries, governments, orphanage administrators, or the bureaucrats pushing the paperwork through. I wanted to feel good about the agency I worked with, but their requirements for adoptive parents included religious affiliation, and they rejected applicants who were openly homosexual. This was typical in the eighties.

I had to ask single applicants why they hadn't married. If they had a roommate of the same gender, I had to ask them to describe that relationship. I didn't have a choice about these questions, but I did have a choice about my response—I accepted their answers. If they were willing to pretend, so was I. But I didn't like working for an agency whose values didn't mesh with mine. And, though I sometimes worked with families who had roots in the country they were adopting from, the majority of adoptive couples were white and financially well-off. These weren't the clients I'd imagined having when I decided to be a social worker. I also had concerns about the long-term adjustment of children placed in families that didn't share their culture or ethnicity.

There were notable exceptions, times when the state contracted with our agency to place US children with families, often minority families because the children needing placement were usually minorities. Once a young Black woman chose our agency to find a family for her child. I worked with her throughout her pregnancy, was at her side for the birth, and supported her after the placement. But her baby stayed in foster care for months while we searched for a family that could afford to cover the costs of prenatal care and delivery.

The fate of this child weighed on me every day until he was placed with his adoptive family. Because of our difficulty in finding an adoptive home, the birth mom indicated some regret about her decision. Her motivation to place her child was largely financial, but those concerns seemed abstract when compared to the essential need of an infant for a mother. While she was pregnant, I had spoken to her about alternatives. I didn't want her to place her child because of the lack of money, but she convinced me adoption was the right plan for her, and I respected her right to make that decision—client autonomy.

Autonomy is the freedom to make your own choices. But her options were meager. I felt too much a part of a system I didn't trust and could not influence.

Having a management position in the ER would mean an opportunity to influence a tiny part of a different system. I would receive additional benefits, most importantly that crucial health insurance at a lower cost. I would be part of a team. I took the promotion and phased out my work with adoptive families. I came to the ER full-time, as the hospital's first ER case manager. I became part of the ER's management team, participating in weekly meetings and administrative decisions. I gave voice to the priorities and challenges of ER advocates and endeavored to support them individually.

I oversaw the hiring and training of advocates, reviewed policies, and created new ones. We built alliances with organizations in our community and increased our knowledge about available services for our patients. I was in the sweet spot of a rare career opportunity born of a creative director's vision and her belief in me and the work.

This was a step toward the ER providing more than Band-Aid care. Having advocates based in and dedicated to the ER already made us unique among area hospitals, but having a social work manager was an even bigger step forward. Our director was eyeing the trends of the big hospital systems, often those outside of the South.

I continued to work a few shifts in the ER, but with other advocates covering most of those shifts, the remainder of my time was spent on a myriad of tasks, including producing yearly staff education modules on social issues hospitals must comply with, such as responding to domestic violence and reporting abuse, and engaging with community agencies. My position became a bountiful catch-all, mirroring my interests and strengths. I felt a surge of professional growth.

One of the primary tasks of my new role was to find and contact patients who needed more help connecting to follow-up care. Diverting those patients to other resources, like primary care or a free clinic, would provide them with preventative care and would help unclog ER flow.

When technology provided a way to get data on the visit history of patients, we saw the problem of ER usage in its enormity. I expected to find the same "frequent flyer" patients making dozens of visits a year. We found that, but we also found that in any three-month period more than fifty patients came to the ER three times or more. Some of those fifty would repeat in a different quarter, but mostly we had a different fifty every quarter.

Doctors and staff clamored for follow-up with our most frequent repeater patients. This was understandable, as they were the biggest users of our limited resources and were often difficult to deal with. You could finish your shift with one of these patients only to see them come in at the start of your next shift. Staff moaned, "Can't case management do something?"

To create our case management program, I reviewed the literature on what other hospitals were doing. Some of the bigger ERs had social workers whose interventions weren't confined to the hospital. They not only connected patients with resources and set up appointments for them, but they also drove them to those appointments. With these extensive interventions, they must have gotten a much clearer view of the obstacles their patients faced. Anything less than this level of commitment seemed unlikely to work with the patients most entrenched in ER usage, but we didn't have funding for that level of advocacy.

There are programs outside of hospitals that operate with this high level of involvement for their clients. I knew of just one such program in our community, run by the county mental health center. I was usually unsuccessful in getting that program to accept our patients because it was underfunded—they didn't have enough staff to take on additional clients. Once they had a client enrolled, the client seemed to stay in the program unless they moved or died. These clients were receiving intensive one-on-one help because nothing else had worked.

There are also stellar individuals working in social service organizations who will make intensive efforts with their client population, but they reserve those efforts for the patients who have not burned bridges, demonstrate a willingness to seek resources or treatment, and (yes, I know how this sounds) *comply* with recommendations. In other words, they will help patients who give some indication that they want help and will follow instructions. This description did not fit our frequent ER users, including Paula.

Paula, the diabetic patient I met when we were both twenty-eight, had never stopped coming to the ER for intoxication and/or syncope related to her diabetes (with intoxication). Now we were thirty-nine.

My son, who was about to start kindergarten when I took the ER job, was now learning to drive. We'd lived in the house my husband built for a decade, enjoying the small neighborhood where we had a group of friends whose children grew up with ours. I played on a tennis team, and my husband started biking. After my father-in-law died, my mother-in-law moved to town, depending on us for groceries, appointments, and companionship. We were busy with full, rich lives; our main complaint was that our jobs were too demanding for time away.

What had these eleven years brought Paula? As far as I knew, nothing had changed for her. She still had untreated diabetes, she still drank too much, and she still got brought in by ambulance and wanted to leave as soon as she arrived.

Now that I was in a new role, could I do more for her? I leaned into the usual discharge instructions: follow-up resources for her drinking and care of her diabetes. She had no desire to stop drinking but didn't overtly object to the recommendation to see someone for her diabetes.

I contacted a community clinic. This is called a "warm referral." Instead of just handing Paula a number with a vague promise that someone would see her, I called the clinic, verified Paula's eligibility to be seen there, and found a manager to be Paula's contact person—Paula could ask for her by name.

But Paula would have to make that call. I did not take the further step of scheduling her appointment because I did not want to burn my bridge with the clinic. I would go out on that limb for the patients who were eager for help and didn't have a decade-long history of not following aftercare recommendations. I didn't need to be begged, thanked, or even appreciated, but Paula didn't show any sign of wanting this referral. I hoped her desire to feel better would overcome any dislike she had for me.

She didn't verbalize any intention to follow up, but she nodded and took the paper from me with the information about the clinic. I was just another person telling her what to do. I wasn't her ally, wasn't someone she could trust. We hadn't built up the mutual regard essential for facilitating change.

Usually in social work when someone is "resistant" (another word I detest), they do at some point at least ask for help. But Paula just woke up and found herself in the ER—she didn't ask to come, and she certainly did not ask me for my help or even my opinion. Yet here I was giving it to her, over and over.

So, the next time she came in with the same problems, I went home with her.

$$\triangle$$

In all my years with the ER, I left the hospital campus with a patient only three times. The first time was after midnight, to help a family retrieve a car seat from their wrecked vehicle, which had been towed to an auto yard. They'd come in by ambulance and were passing through town to a nearby state. The accident had been minor, and everyone checked out OK, but the person coming to get them had no car seat for the infant.

Security wasn't available to come with me. They were shorthanded late at night and couldn't spare personnel to go off campus. I drove the father of the infant to the auto yard in my car. It wasn't far, and everyone knew where I was going; still, it felt like a very bad idea even as I did it. But it was the only idea I had—the only way to have some assurance of the infant's safety and to prevent the family being delayed in the ER hours longer than necessary.

I could have waited for the person coming to get them to obtain a car seat or take the father to get one. But that assumed they had money to buy one, and besides, no store was open. Their friend wasn't due for hours, and I was already past the end of my shift, with no one scheduled to come after me. I was exhausted and due back in twelve hours. The family had been discharged; they were no longer our patients in anyone's eyes but mine.

In later years, the roles of charge nurses and nurse managers would evolve to include supporting the advocates as needed in problem-solving, whether the issue was medical or social. There would often be two advocates working at the same time so that they could help each other. And we'd have an advocate on call, or, in my position as manager, I could be contacted with such problems.

But none of that existed at this time, and I couldn't stand to make this family's ordeal worse when I could be part of a solution that got them out and on their way. I also didn't trust the family not to just get in the car when their ride came, and skip the auto yard altogether, putting the child in the car with no car seat. Or, if they went to get the car seat, I wasn't sure they could get in the auto yard without me. I'd negotiated this visit with the night shift tow truck driver, who was reluctant to allow them in their vehicle without payment. The family couldn't pay.

Nothing bad happened. I drove the father there and back without incident and got the car seat. Once a car seat is in an accident, it needs to be inspected before it's used again, or preferably, it's replaced. I was not qualified to inspect it and unable to replace it. I could only see that it was in place in the wrecked car, seemingly intact, with all the straps working. I advised them to get a new seat or have this one checked out, and they played their part, assuring me they would.

By leaving the hospital I'd broken boundaries, my employers' and my own. I felt betrayed—like it was the hospital's fault that I was placed in a vulnerable situation. I went home and slept a few hours, returning the next day for another twelve-hour shift. The day shift charge nurse heard about this field trip of mine and scolded me for putting myself at risk, saying, "I wouldn't have let you do that." I was both offended and comforted.

She was the kind of charge nurse we would have in the future—one with an expansive view of risk and a willingness to take on issues beyond standard patient care. If she had been working that night, we would have found a different solution.

The last time I left the hospital with a patient, it was to ensure a young woman with mental health issues had a safe place to go. The mental health worker based in the ER, who was inundated with patients needing admission, said the patient could be discharged if we could verify her home situation; they would not release her "to the street." She had no visitors and had no one for me to call. She insisted she was staying in a home nearby.

Security could take her and asked me to ride as an escort. We went to the address she gave us. The door was locked. She didn't have a key but assured us she knew a way in, striding toward a side window. I glanced at the security guard, and we scurried after her, protesting loudly that this was not a good idea. She was already on top of a garbage can.

This was perilous and possibly illegal. Should we hold the garbage can for her or pull her off of it? We conferred in a panic—was it better to help her or prevent her? Did we have the right to do either?

She knew just how to jimmy that window; she was inside in no time. What if she got hurt? We ran to the window and yelled, "Are you OK?" She answered that she was fine, thanks for the ride. We shook our heads at all the ways that could have gone bad for each of us and remained uncertain about leaving her. But we were tasked with bringing her here, she said this was where she stayed, and she was now inside. We left.

The ER was the devil we knew—full of its own risks but with a clear blueprint and a team of coworkers. Outside was a slippery world where our roles blurred, where we didn't know how to keep patients safe, or how to keep ourselves safe with them.

In the years before my promotion, I considered leaving the ER to become a hospice social worker. With adoptions, I'd worked in the homes of growing families starting new chapters. Hospice work would put me at the opposite end of the lifespan. I could apply what I'd learned about changes in family systems with adoptions, augmented with what I knew about grief from the ER. There was no sugarcoating hospice. That appealed to me.

But the ER had already worked its curse on me. Now that I knew how randomly unsafe the world was, the thought of taking my work on the road was disturbing. I'd grown dependent on the familiarity of working within a structure I understood—the ER was the home I knew. I needed that familiarity to face the unfamiliar, some predictability to balance the chaos of unpredictability.

△

Although they never rode in with her, we knew Paula had family because we'd call them to take her home once she was sober. Her aunts, or someone they called, came and got her. This time I decided we would take her home.

She confirmed she lived close by, and family was there. She gave me permission to talk to her family about her medical issues. Security staff drove us to an ordinary, comfortable-seeming apartment that gave no clue that someone living there got brought to the ER on a regular basis. Her family seemed kind and warm; they welcomed me.

They listened to me lay out her need for regular care and were familiar with the clinic I had called. They were willing to try, but they made no guarantees. "Paula's gonna do what Paula's gonna do." Paula sat by in sullen silence. It didn't matter how much we wanted this for her if she didn't want it for herself.

Still, I was naive enough to be hopeful. I gave her aunts my card and the clinic information. I got their numbers and called them when Paula's visits increased. They had set up appointments for her at the clinic, but she wouldn't go. We continued to see her once or twice a month in the ER, sometimes more, sometimes less, usually worse.

My initial case management efforts were focused on patients like Paula. When those patients came to the ER, a physician often set the tone of the visit, either "nice ER" or "mean ER," in our futile attempts to effect behavioral change. Our carrots were cafeteria sandwiches and bus vouchers, exchanged for a patient's agreement to follow up with the appropriate resource. Our sticks were few: the absence of any frills, "no extras," such as a warm blanket or cold soda, as ordered by the doctor. Stern lectures were given about ER usage. But even the most frequent patient with the most frustrating behavior was assessed medically each time we saw them, even if they came every day for a week.

We knew these patients for years. Most of them had long-standing mental health diagnoses and/or a history of addiction, along with chronic illnesses. They had poor or nonexistent social supports, and they were accustomed to coming to the ER. We could ask about their needs and obstacles and factor that into our recommendations, but in the end, we were still just telling them what to do from our perspective. This is what we do in health care.

As social work manager, I dove into the list of these frequent users, reviewed their charts, came up with resources, and made calls. I often couldn't reach the patients by phone, so I sent them letters with my number and kept my eye out for those names to show up on our electronic tracking board of current patients. If they returned when I was there, I met with them in person. At least then I knew whether they had received the resources I sent, and I could give them my number again so they could contact me in the future.

Because in-person meetings required the luck of perfect timing and therefore didn't happen often, I made my recommendations available to the other advocates so they could pass on this information when the patient visited during their shift. Not surprisingly, an additional contact by me or another advocate did not make a difference to our most frequent patients. I might not see them or hear of their visits, but every time I ran the data, there they were—their names topping the list with the highest number of visits. Nevertheless, I had to try multiple times with each of those patients in order to convince staff that my failures were not from a lack of effort or intention. There was an expectation that referring a patient for case management would "fix" them, as if I had a magic wand. What drove patients to make repeated ER visits was a combination of desperation, a lack of an accessible alternative, and/or an entrenched personal habit. Lasting solutions would require intensive interventions with community-wide services.

I turned my focus to new patients making multiple visits, the ones whose names we didn't know yet and who might be receptive to my help. I found plenty of patients with new problems, diagnoses, or injuries that required follow-up they'd been unable to receive for a variety of reasons.

Many of these patients welcomed assistance navigating the medical system, and I used the reduction of their visits as proof that what I did mattered, though I had to face down my own doubts each day. These patients didn't come often enough for staff to miss them, to notice that they weren't there. I may have made a difference in their lives, but that didn't translate to a tangible difference in the lives of the ER staff.

Doing this work took me out of the trenches of direct immediate care. Recognizing my contributions as a team member required imagination on the part of staff. The daily reality for staff was that the work was extremely hard and getting harder all the time.

I reached for ways that my actions could make a difference. Imagination was now a waste of time.

We May Not Let You Die, but You Are Free to Suffer

When I was told by hospital administration that there wasn't a reporting form for elder abuse because "We don't see any of that," I created the form because I was seeing plenty of that.

Most elder reports made are for "self-neglect." Their blood pressure is untreated despite having an ongoing prescription, or they have diabetes and are not eating well. They may have been brought to the ER due to the worsening of these conditions, an injury from a fall, or reports that they've been wandering, lost in their own neighborhood.

Usually, these patients arrive by ambulance, and medics paint a dire picture of the home. We hear about places that lack air conditioning or heat, are filled with bugs, have empty or broken refrigerators, or have so much clutter that there are only rabbit paths from room to room through stacks of paper or piles of clothes and trash, creating a fire hazard. The medic tells me emphatically that we can't let them return home. I nod my head.

I don't have the heart to tell them that the patient will almost certainly go back home, and I don't have the time to explain why. Soon enough the medic will discover that conditions they find deplorable, that they believe are inconsistent with the most minimal quality of life, are considered "good enough" by our culture. They saw the patient living in a way they didn't think existed in this country. They wouldn't tolerate any of their relatives living like that, and they can't imagine anyone else tolerating it. But people live in conditions that defy imagination, sometimes because they cannot stomach the alternatives.

While we care for the patient and wait on test results, we call relatives, neighbors, anyone we can find through information on the chart
or by piecing together numbers and names that the patient has tucked
into their pockets or purse or can dimly recall. Our quest is to find
someone who can make things better for the patient by picking up
their medicine, helping them pay their electric bill, taking them to a
follow-up appointment. If there's not a medical reason for admission,
the patient will be sent back, regardless of horrible conditions in the
home and how compromised their health is.

There is the occasional exception: a "social admission" for patients in extreme situations. Social admissions rarely happened when
I started in the ER and may not ever happen now. When a patient did
not have a medical condition that required admission but absolutely
could not go home, they were admitted for social reasons. It was to be
avoided at all costs—because of the cost. Insurance, if the patient had
it, demanded a medical reason for admission, and hospitals could not
afford to eat that bill. It made the hospital look like the bad guy, but
communities and entire regions suffer when a hospital goes bankrupt.
A closed hospital serves no one. Medical resources should be used
for medical issues, but we have failed to build adequate safety nets
for those in free fall from anything not meeting hospital admission
criteria.

When we made a report to adult protective services, social workers from that county department would visit the patient at home.
They'd assess the patient's needs and offer various resources, including
housing. A daily delivery of lunch might sound appealing, but they'd
have to outlive those on the waiting list ahead of them before they
could enjoy a single meal. Perhaps they'd be eligible for a home aide
to help with basic care and housekeeping, but that also came with a
long wait and let a stranger into their home at a time when they might
feel vulnerable and self-conscious, if not ashamed, of their home and
situation.

These patients would make another visit to the ER. The medic who
brought them in last time would be stunned to find the patient still in
that home, in worse shape than before. They'd confront me: How did

I let this happen? Didn't I understand? Didn't I believe them? I'd tell them that I tried to get the patient admitted, and when that failed, I made a report.

Once a medic pulled me into a room to meet Mr. Hughes, an elderly patient they'd just brought in. Confined to a wheelchair, he no longer had the strength to transfer himself to his bed or the bathroom. He lived alone in his own home. Mr. Hughes called the medics regularly, but I had never met him because he always refused transport to the hospital, having only called them to assist him with some "minor" need, like going to the bathroom or obtaining food.

The wheelchair was an electric one, its seat shredded because he was living in it. He ate the one meal a day that was delivered and he never went to the doctor. He would not agree to move to a facility because the only thing he owned was his house and he was saving it for his son, who was in prison. If he left his house for a facility, it would be sold to pay for his room and board. His son would have nothing.

But now the wheelchair was broken, and even the most basic makeshift maneuvers—getting to the fridge, sink, or toilet's lever to flush his urine or feces—were impossible. So, he called the ambulance. All he wanted them to do was clean him up. They insisted on bringing him in. All he wanted me to do was get his wheelchair fixed. The doctor examined him, but admission wasn't discussed because the patient refused to consider it.

I called the medical device company that provided maintenance on the chair. They said the chair malfunctioned because it wasn't meant to be lived in. They had cleaned it and repaired it before. A new chair would not be covered by Medicare. They grudgingly agreed to loan him a chair while they took his in to again clean and repair it. We sent him home. I made a report. He called the ambulance the next week but refused transport. The medic came and found me.

The patient's county social worker in adult protective services confirmed that my report was received. They had met with the patient. Services and options were presented, and he declined everything except the meal delivery. The social worker had no reason to return to his home—their client, our patient, had made his choice.

I'm sure there were times when the worker responded to our report, met the elder patient in their home, and the elder accepted help and didn't come back to the ER. I wouldn't know about those patients, because those were best-case scenarios, and I worked in the realm of the opposite.

In my early years at the ER, I went to see our employee health services for a cyst on my thigh. A surgeon working there that day gave me his card. He said such cysts never resolved and I would have to have it surgically removed. I didn't make an appointment immediately, suspecting that the surgeon suffered from the same affliction I had—a perversion of perception. He only saw the cases that didn't resolve and assumed that his normal was *the* normal. Within a few weeks, my cyst was gone with no further intervention. The surgeon had erroneously generalized his unique experience to the world beyond, where, it turns out, plenty of people have cysts that don't require surgery.

Similarly, I cannot know the true scope of the problem of self-neglect because I saw only one side, and it was where the ideal of patient autonomy rubbed raw against the fantasy that we take care of people in this country. If we hold the value of independence so highly, then why don't we have more options to help our elders stay safely independent as long as possible?

△

For the elderly or disabled living in facilities, there is a different process of reporting and response. Instead of problem and risk assessment with resource linking, the focus is on facility compliance with standards of care.

The first time an ER director called me in to discuss a report, she explained that she'd received a call from our irate hospital administrator, who'd had a call from a furious nursing home director. My director explained that my report of neglect (lack of blood pressure checks and timely medication in a hypertensive patient) sent to a state agency charged with nursing home supervision prompted an unannounced visit by inspectors. I think she expected me to be shocked and horrified that a report from little ol' me, a lowly social worker, could have such an outsized impact, could ignite such a significant action. It's true that this was more than I had expected . . . and I was delighted. Finally, a process I could admire! Potential risk taken seriously, and an immediate response launched.

A report prompting an unannounced official visit sounded reasonable to me, but hospital administrators know the stress of scrutiny and what happens when a state agency tasked with compliance makes a visit. Investigators can look anywhere and cite the facility for anything. Fines often result, as well as damage to reputation. An improvement process is outlined that takes staff time and resources away from patients and means additional visits from inspectors to check on progress, which can result in more findings. A facility can stay trapped in that loop for months or longer. But that's how a place improves, right? To ensure that changes are made to make things better for the residents? A facility responsible for caring for others must be held accountable for its deficits.

Administrators were concerned with community relationships, including the nursing homes in the area, who help us decompress a full hospital by expediting acceptance and transfer of a patient that no longer needs hospital care but doesn't have anywhere else to go. The nursing homes need our business, and we need their help. To then turn around and sic the state investigators on them was contrary to good business and Southern manners. My report blindsided the hospital administrator and put my director in the hot seat.

I always thought that this was the issue that would cause me to leave, because it bumped up against a line I wouldn't cross. Not making a report when a patient is significantly harmed or at risk to be harmed, through action or inaction, would be an ethical and moral violation on my part, one I couldn't live with. If I felt a report needed to be made, I was going to make it. If anyone prevented me from doing so, then I would report them as well.

Three different ER directors dealt with me over this issue during my career. Each sheltered me from hospital administrators highly annoyed by those calls from nursing home administrators. Thankfully my directors were all nurses. They understood that the patient's welfare was more important than the embarrassment of hospital top brass. Each time a director called me in to ask me about a report, I knew the report had triggered a reaction from on high. I made it clear that I would leave over this issue, and each time they talked me down. They didn't disregard my advocacy or concerns, but they recognized that these reports were made in the chaos of the moment. A cleaner process would help the directors defend our reports.

Part of the problem was time. Reports were too problematic to routinely hand off. On a busy shift an advocate might stay late to complete one and still not have all the pertinent details. We might still be waiting for test results or X-rays, or for a call back from a family member or the medic who transported the patient. But the advocate who met the patient and initiated the report might not be back on shift for days. There was an obligation for the advocate who received information—whether from medical staff, family members, or the patient themselves—to ensure the ER took appropriate action.

When hearing about atrocities from an eyewitness or a medical provider at the bedside, there's a visceral response that gets lost or diluted in subsequent telling. This physical connection is what carries you through the hard work of reporting: hunting down details, filling out paperwork, contacting agencies, often staying late for those test results or to get through on the phone to confirm that the report was received. When your shift relief arrives, you could hand off completion of the report. But each advocate applied their own litmus test to those situations. They weren't going to make a report "just" because their coworker felt like one should be made—they were going to make their own assessment with the information that would now be secondhand. It seems like a betrayal of professional collaboration to not accept the baton from your colleague and run it over the finish line by completing the report, but in addition to the critically divisive mindset so often present in ER team members, there is a practical consideration.

Reports can result in a court case. Whoever completed the report could be called to testify. No one wants to state on the stand that they made a report only because someone asked them to. People's lives and businesses can be destroyed from a report, because our reports are taken seriously, hence we have a professional obligation to report out of a compulsion of duty to the patient—not duty to a colleague.

Once an advocate determines a report is warranted, if they delay reporting, they could be liable for the consequences. In my new position, I was in the ER most weekdays. Information from a night shift could be left for me to supplement a few hours later with test results or a medic's report. I could contact the investigating agency during weekday hours. If I didn't feel there was a clear reason to report, then I would contact the advocate. They could always come in and do the report themselves if so inclined, but usually I trusted their judgment and followed through on making the report they recommended. As a manager, I assumed that hypothetical court would understand that I couldn't always be on the front lines, but I had an obligation to those frontline workers, stemming from a shared mission to keep patients safe.

On average, we made one report each week of either child or elder abuse or neglect. Most of the elder reports regarded patients living in their own homes. Given the thousand or so patients we saw in a week, reporting such concerns was not a frequent duty, but it was one of our most important.

I was never discouraged from making a report, even when it concerned a facility that was sure to push back. I was, however, encouraged to see the full picture. We weren't held to absolute certainty about our reports but were encouraged to decrease subjectivity by increasing our information.

When reporting a facility, we tightened our process to include a more thorough review, including more involvement from the physician who saw the patient, as they could better evaluate the impact of care (or lack of care). When the concern regarded something low risk, like incomplete or missing medical documentation, our ER director would call the nursing home director and have a nurse-to-nurse conversation. If the issue was not medical, such as a complaint about

staff or allegation of theft, we worked with our region's ombudsmen—
community liaisons who follow up with care facilities in a cooperative
relationship.

Working with the facilities in this way did not have to mean a
reduction in protection for their residents. Advocates reported as
needed, skipping the physician review if the concern was clearly serious and urgent, like allegations of abuse by nursing home staff or
other residents. My instinct for a fight fizzled under the modulating
influence of ER directors. There was still a line in the sand, but up
to that line were new options. I recognized a characteristic in myself,
something that thrilled to the idea of quitting a job under protest.

When I was a teenager taking some absolute stance with my
mother, she called me self-righteous. I had never heard that term, so I
looked it up. She wasn't wrong. Before I left home, I became an outspo-
ken vegetarian, confronted classmates when they uttered racial slurs,
and skirted holiday meal preparations, because this only fell to the
women while the men relaxed. When I went to college, I plastered my
car with anti-nuke bumper stickers.

I wanted it known that if my ethics were tested, I would act. I
would emerge with my principles intact even if it meant losing my job.

But who was I trying to convince?

Please Schedule Your Emergency

The ER is busier during the holidays because doctors' offices are closed. Certain hospital departments may also close, leaving ER staff to smirk. *"It must be nice."* If only emergencies could be scheduled, then we could do that. But the ER never closes. I've worked in places with long hours—libraries, hotels, Shoney's—but 24/7 for 365 is entirely different. There are no holidays. There are various ways to divide up shifts falling on holidays, and none of them are fair. They all result in each staff member having to work some hours that they'd rather spend with family. The needs of the ER are relentless, and they devour the lives of those who work there, disregarding even once-in-a-lifetime moments, such as graduations and weddings.

Calling out sick on a holiday is assumed to be a ploy, and savvy managers counter this with a requirement to work the next holiday when the worker was scheduled off. If you're legitimately sick on Christmas Day, come in and prove it. Witnessed vomiting usually gets you excused. Technically, a fever during flu season should bar you from working, but it depends on how many staff already called out.

None of us like the idea of working holidays, but once there, it's usually a better-than-average day to work. For one thing, there's free food. In addition to staff and doctors bringing in food to share, ERs are often recipients of food from generous community groups and restaurants. Sometimes a meal in the cafeteria is free. Usually, the pace of the ER is too hectic to allow you to get to the cafeteria, but holidays offer ER workers a chance to experience this bit of normalcy that most hospital staff take for granted.

I usually worked Christmas Day, and preferred the years it fell on a weekend, so that I worked with my old team, the Baylor staff. On that Baylor staff was Brian. A paramedic before he became a nurse, Brian was one of my favorite nurses. He radiated compassion, but if pushed by a patient's behavior or a doctor's demands, he calmly but tenaciously stood his ground. I never saw him flustered. On Christmas, he brought us treats. One year he handed out scarves he'd hand-woven for the staff. Another year he made flavored seasonings and put them in small glass bottles of red and green.

Each Christmas he worked, he brought a leather collar of bells, the kind that horses wear in snowy Christmas commercials. He would go to the inpatient units at mealtimes and ask permission of the charge nurses before donning the bells and a Santa hat. Then he would run up and down the hallways, filling them with a robust festive jingle. I pictured the patients in their beds along those corridors. How curious it must have been to hear distant bells getting nearer, then loud as he passed their door, then softer again. A sensory pause in the tedium, isolation, and pain of a hospital stay. How wonderful that someone would go to that trouble to give others a moment of delight.

Another nice thing about working a holiday is that administrators aren't around. Their absence, along with the plentiful food, evokes a celebratory vibe—a break in the routine. Best of all, it's usually not busy, because no patients want to come in. You might think this is a given every day, that no one ever *wants* to come to the ER, but it doesn't seem that way to those of us working there, except on holidays.

Halloween is a normal busy day until late afternoon, when the ER empties out as trick-or-treating starts. But, after darkness falls, people and cars mingle, and accidents increase. I worked many Halloweens before the hospital put the kibosh on staff dressing up. Staff in costume makes even a nontraumatic visit too bizarre and undermines the professional image.

Banning costumes is one of those administrative decisions that the staff groans about—a prime example, they'll say, of the hospital going too "corporate." Even if the staff steered away from scary or offensive costume choices, do you really want your blood pressure taken by someone wearing cat ears or a needle stuck in your arm by a clown? Picture Raggedy Ann intubating a patient in respiratory distress and then going to speak to the family. How can a freakish doll establish credibility? It smears an extra layer of surrealism onto an experience that is already surreal enough.

The bigger the holiday is, the fewer patients we have, but those patients we do have are often sicker than usual. Those injured only come in if X-rays or sutures are needed, and sick patients delay coming until their condition worsens or even becomes critical.

△

In the 1934 movie *Death Takes a Holiday*, Death is a character who comes to Earth as a human. While he's here, no one dies. Apparently, he is shirking his responsibilities while discovering what the human experience of living is all about.

We'd like him to sync his holiday with our holidays. There are days when no one dies in the ER, so is it really too much to ask that no one die on a major holiday? Holiday deaths are harder on everyone. The family has to reconcile the memory of trauma and loss with an occasion that is joyous for others and was once joyous for them. For the staff, the survivor guilt is heavier than usual—we carry the memory of others' losses into our future holidays.

Each Christmas, I recall the family who had just sat down for their festive meal when the matriarch went into cardiac arrest. They filled our Family Room as we did compressions and later pronounced her. The doctor was new to the ER, and it was my first time working a death with him.

Working with a new doctor brings extra stress, especially if this is their first death in your ER. No one knows their style: Will they delay talking with the family, preferring instead to immerse themselves into a new case? Some doctors like to switch gears immediately, shake off what might feel like a failure. I had gleaned these insights by turning to nurses in my frustration. They seemed to understand better than I did what the doctor may be personally confronting while the family hung in limbo. I sat with those families, wordlessly willing the doctor to come in, even as I dreaded what would follow. Part of my preparation at such times came from knowing what to expect from the physician, knowing their script. I had no idea what this new doctor would say or how he would say it.

Turned out, the new doctor had his routine down and it was a good one. He came in promptly, introduced himself, sat down with them, and gave a very brief review of the course of treatment: "She arrived without a heartbeat, so we did CPR, which is heart compressions." He made the motions with his hands. Then he made the turn: "Unfortunately her heart did not start beating again. She died. I'm sorry." He stayed. He waited quietly, taking cues from the family and from me, offering to come back and talk to them if they had questions.

I went to check the room before bringing in the family and found the nurse wide-eyed. The patient had resumed breathing. It's not that unusual to have agonal breathing: breaths that do not produce enough oxygen to feed the brain or heart and continue for a short while. But her breaths continued much longer than usual. We called the doctor into the room. This went beyond his experience as well.

He asked the nurse to hook her back up to a monitor and gave me a wild look, knowing what I represented—the burden of having to go back into that Family Room to try to tell a new truth, one harder, possibly, even than death, because what does a family do with this information? I met his gaze and confirmed his fear: "We have to tell them, but what do we say?"

The impact this would have on the family was unpredictable. They were waiting to see her. We couldn't bring them in unprepared, nor could we leave them waiting without explanation, even though the explanation might make us look incompetent or give them false hope. The patient was not going to revive; this was just a postponement of the inevitable.

Now I would really see what this new doctor was made of. As he and the nurse and I stood awkwardly next to the barely but persistently breathing patient, we were gathering courage. I believe I was the most nervous. Given my professional training, my time spent in the ER, and my age (the oldest in the room, not counting the patient), I probably knew the most about human nature and how sideways this could go. And I was still uncertain of this doctor—how would he navigate this new territory?

In a tension-relieving gesture, he shrugged, managing his own apprehension, finding his matter-of-fact professional demeanor as he practiced it on me: This was uncommon but not unheard of. The patient would be monitored, and if she continued to breathe, we would admit her. Not for medical interventions, he carefully added, but so the family could remain at her bedside and be in a more comfortable and private location.

I wouldn't blame any family for seeing this as a miracle. I've seen families stand and pray over bodies unquestionably dead, certain that God would perform a resurrection. This family could accuse us of stopping treatment too soon. There were many ways this could go terribly wrong.

The doctor went to the family wearing his most humble persona. He got the words out despite their impossibility. He reminded them that her heart had stopped and would not restart. Her breathing had stopped . . . but then resumed. He explained that agonal breathing is a reflex of the body but is unproductive, the breaths coming only occasionally. They would soon stop again. We would not be doing any further interventions. He wanted them to be prepared if they heard her breathe as they stood by her bed. The family took this in calmly.

There are many beliefs among medical staff that I don't buy into, but the belief that a patient often "waits" to die seems real to me. The patient had been separated from her family during her ER treatment, but as they now sat beside her and told her goodbye, her breathing slowly stopped. I had wished they didn't have this strange circumstance to complicate their loss, but they found meaning in it.

I may be guilty of exploiting the thinnest places for evidence of spirit over matter. Experiences not easily dissected by facts are, to me, an invitation to consider something more. I want that space for wonder. I want to believe that our Christmas Day patient, who was probably rule abiding in life, stubbornly refused in death to comply with our routine.

At some point in every code I was part of, somewhere between compressions and pronouncement, I turned my eyes up to the ceiling.

Patients who survive a code sometimes say that their spirits lingered above the staff bent over their dying bodies. I worried about the patients' aloneness—their spirits up there, watching us all together below, our heads bent down, looking for them in bodies they were now separate from, everyone looking for them in the wrong place. I don't assume such reports of near-death experiences are true, but neither can I dismiss them.

I was the only one who had the time, and perhaps the inclination, to do this in the midst of the code. No one expected me to start a line, do compressions, document on a chart, or push medicine. Looking up, I offered my hope for the path that was right for them—the way back or the way out.

The worst-case scenario was that I was foolish, but the best-case scenario was that these actions mattered, if only to me, and that's what kept me doing it. The worst-case scenario does not triumph every time even in the ER, and I was accustomed to seeming foolish in the eyes of my peers. Though some of them may not have thought this was foolish at all—a nurse once told me that as she did compressions on a trauma patient, she felt her spirit pass right through her.

△

We moved out of the old ER once we had a section of the new one built. On moving day, after all the staff had ferried supplies and patients out to the new unit and the workmen had filed in with tools of destruction, I went back for a final look. The old space would eventually be integrated into our new, larger department, but first it would be demolished, never again recognizable as the space I knew, the space where I saw so many patients die.

That old ER was itself dead—silent, empty, and dim. The air felt heavy with lives, including those of the coworkers who had died during those years, inside or outside the ER: a longtime charge nurse known for his snarky observations but tender heart; two unit secretaries—one young and sharp, who died soon after moving away to build a new life, and the other a longtime employee who kept us laughing at his hilarious impressions of all the doctors; and a nurse in her forties, who was the best the profession had to offer, lighting up every room she walked into, giving excellent care.

As I stood in that old ER, remembering them, I didn't think about the deaths to come, of patients and staff. Three beloved nurses who made that move from the old to the new ER would die young from various cancers. Cancer would also take a housekeeper whose gentle spirit graced our department for many years. One of the advocates worked with Habitat for Humanity to get a home for her and her young family, and a group of us gave a day to working on the house. The ER has got to be the worst hospital assignment possible for a housekeeper, but she declined a transfer. She was part of our team.

An older nurse from the Baylor shift, Joan, retired before we left the old ER, before we started electronic charting. I think she suspected how computers would transform nursing, or maybe she just wasn't up for yet another change in a career spanning decades of changes. She was an artist, and one year she painted a banner in appreciation of the advocates. It had a note of thanks in her flowing calligraphy, with flowers around the edges in burgundy and dark blue. When the banner was taken down, I claimed it. My tiny office in the airshaft didn't have a wall long enough to hang it, but my next office did, and the one after that, and the one after that.

Soon after I hung the banner in that last office, we learned that Joan was dying. When I was ready to retire, I knew no one else cherished that banner like I did. I cut it up and framed the painted flowers. One of them sits beside me as I write this.

But I'm making Joan sound sweet, and that isn't fair to her. She was so much more than that. Her kindness came out with patients, but rarely with the staff or doctors. The epitome of the stern older nurse stereotype, Joan was a no-nonsense, hardworking woman who'd stood up for her patients for decades, facing down dismissals of her opinions and experiences. She didn't have time for fluff or pretense. She did not suffer fools.

Once, when a young father interrupted a mother who was describing their child's symptoms, Joan told him to be quiet, he was just "the sperm donor." She regretted it right away, blushed an apology to the dad, and later confessed to our director. She was focused on the sick child and getting the information we needed from the primary caregiver, who was the mom. Joan was sheepish when she told me, realizing she had rudely dismissed that dad. But as far as I knew, no complaint came from it. She had a way of saying things with a twinkle in her eye and a hint of affection.

Joan told me you should ring in the new year by doing what you loved. On New Year's Eve, she stayed up past midnight to paint. I can't match her creative stamina, but her example inspires me to welcome in each first of January by writing.

After Joan retired, we didn't see her again until she came in as a patient. She didn't come back for social visits or parties, or stay in touch by Facebook. She broke clean, diving deep into her life of art and family. I admired her for that and for so much more. She died a few months after I retired. Covid meant no funeral service and no chance for the ER team to reunite and share our stories of her. When I think of her, I see her in that old ER.

"That old ER" had been newly renovated when I started in 1991, and now, about ten years later, it was being rebuilt. I was part of its ten-year lifespan, part of a team that existed in one small segment of time in a hospital's existence. I outlived that old ER, but I'd been rebuilt as well. I took one last look around as the workmen dug in. The patient rooms were all empty. The ER finally closed.

△

By evening, the pause of activity on holidays ends with a vengeance. As the ambulances arrive one after another, staff says, "We're paying for our good day now."

People having too much fun, or too much sorrow when they

expected fun, is a common thread running among patients on the holidays. Family tension brewing all day erupts into violent squabbles fueled by the day's drinking, or family members drive away into accidents, or Grandpa finally admits he's having chest pain.

The day after the holiday brings all the patients who put off their visit. It's a wise move to work the holiday shift and take off the day after, but good luck explaining that to your family.

That Christmas when the matriarch died in her own time, the new doctor stopped by my desk on his way out. "And now, I get to go home and have dinner with my family," he said ruefully. He knew it wasn't fair—that he had an intact family waiting for him to eat a celebratory meal together. This experience went home with him, and perhaps, like me, it joins him at the table every Christmas.

I nodded at him that day in shared understanding and told him to enjoy that dinner. What passed between us was unsaid: We knew each other now in the only way that mattered in the ER world—we could depend on each other when things got sad and strange. We both knew that life is a gift that can end on any day of the week, even a holiday.

Sins of Omission

As with mortal sins, mistakes in the profession of social work are usually acts of commission or omission: things done or things left undone. I worried most about errors of omission.

When social workers fail to see or understand something about a situation, the consequences for a vulnerable person can be severe. Perhaps they fail to read the dynamic between a patient and her spouse—indicators that she's under his control. The signs can be as mild as her looking at him before she talks or as bold as his insistence to be present for the pelvic exam.

The omission could be not seeing the large plastic bag lying under the gurney, all the possessions the patient couldn't risk leaving behind in the car he's living in. Or in failing to realize that the elderly woman with no visitors does indeed have family—they dropped her off with a phone number they don't answer for hours—yet no one in the ER asks her about her homelife.

It's impossible to meet every patient, but advocates keep an eye on computer tracking boards. Before we had those, we hunted down paper charts, often finding them in the dark corners of the tiny dictation room, stashed there by doctors to ensure they would be handy when they had the time to review and document.

Electronic charting has its downsides. Nurses, nurse practitioners, physician assistants, and doctors say it changed the way they practice, and no one who said that ever meant that the change was an improvement. They don't like the way it pivots their focus from the patient beside them to a computer screen with boxes that demand checking. Because protocols are built into the system, checking certain boxes prompts new questions and boxes that suggest tests and treatments with which the provider—having the benefit of seeing and touching the patient beside them—may not agree. It can lead a provider down a road of "rule-outs" that they otherwise would not have taken.

But if you've been seen at the ER before or by a medical system that we have access to, we have your medical information at our fingertips. This can save your life or allow us to find the blood pressure medication whose name you can't remember and that you ran out of on Christmas Eve when your pharmacy was closed. An electronic chart improves efficiency and reduces the time you're stuck in the ER because multiple people can access it at the same time—no more waiting turns.

A person who has never worked in a paper chart world cannot appreciate how very common it was for charts to go missing, how much time was wasted as staff waited or searched, growing increasingly frustrated. The hierarchy of the medical world was reflected in how much time you got with the paper chart. Doctors could batch, stack, hide, or hold them, whereas nurses would take only a moment to sit down with one, documenting as they gulped coffee, and quickly return it to the chart rack. Advocates would chart while standing at the chart rack, not even taking the chart away.

Advocates flipped through charts to suss out red flags from the presenting problem and medical history. But mostly, we relied on nurses, techs, and doctors to report their concerns, as they were present at every bedside. We worried most about missing a sign of possible child abuse. Usually this was evidence of neglect: a condition worsened by delayed medical treatment, or an injury (or accidental overdose) resulting from lack of supervision. If a child was present during a domestic violence incident or a suicide attempt, the ongoing risk to the child may warrant a report.

These are the "easy" cases, because the risk we perceive is not usually significant enough to require an immediate assessment by child protective services for possible removal from the home. Resources are given to the parents, follow-up care explained, and a report made to the county social services. The child can go home with the parent who brought them. Child protective workers will follow up with the family unless they screen out our report. Reports can be screened out for lack of information and/or lack of reasonable apparent risk.

We know that being reported can be a nightmare for the family, but we are bound by professional obligation to report our concerns. Social workers, along with all hospital personnel, first responders, teachers, counselors, and many others, are mandated reporters.

Soon after I started working in the ER, the department's director sent me to a Train the Trainers reporting workshop. She wanted me to expand our training to the entire staff so they could recognize potential abuse and neglect.

Advocates can't be everywhere, and we didn't cover the department around the clock. Nurses and techs are often at the bedside, and in the intimacy of caring for the patient, they see things an advocate never would: physical evidence like bruises, or emotional indicators like a lack of attachment—a parent unconcerned with their child's crying.

I offered the class a couple of times a year until our accrediting organization (a national body who ensured we met certain standards, required for good standing and to receive government money) said that all direct care providers in ERs had to have specific training. I ramped up to get everyone trained before our next accreditation review.

One of the first things I addressed in the class was what keeps us from making a report. The attendees would list the obstacles, all of which were realistic issues: doubting the system, not believing that a report would do any good; a fear of reprisals from the family; not wanting to judge the family; not wanting to burden the family with involvement of authorities. But the most common worry was that we could be wrong, that we didn't have enough information to know a report was warranted. Our training materials said that a mandated reporter is held to a "reasonable concern."

Our job was to identify reasonable concerns about risks to a child.

If the county's protective services determined our reported concerns not to be reasonable, they would screen out those reports.

We kept stats on our reports. Over time, the number screened out came down to a few per year. This means our reports reflected reasonable concerns from the perspective of child protective services. We didn't want to over-report, but the worry of not reporting something you should have gnawed at you, keeping you awake.

△

Another obstacle to making a report is the influence of our peers. When someone comes out of a patient room and describes what they saw, heard, or simply felt, it's easy to dismiss it—you weren't there. We talked in class about being aware of this and the importance of trying to get a sense of what spooked your coworker.

None of us wants to believe that a parent would hurt a child. We want to believe that loving a child precludes such behaviors. Yet those of us who are parents know that we've been at risk of going too far when we lose our temper. I have certainly crossed my own lines of parental standards, yet I never stopped loving my children.

When loving parents brought their one-year-old child in with an injury to her leg, it was diagnosed as a femur fracture. Her parents' story of a short fall down a few steps was questioned. The femur (thigh bone) is the strongest and longest bone in the body. Also, children's bones have some flexibility and do not break easily, unless the child has a medical condition that causes their bones to be brittle. The most likely cause of a femur fracture in a child who isn't walking yet is a car accident, a long fall . . . or abuse.

This fractured femur aroused everyone's suspicions, but a report was not made due to the comfort staff felt with her parents. She was discharged home with her family. Soon afterward, we read about her death in the local paper. She was one of three unrelated children to die from abuse that year in our county. All of them first had femur fractures and were not yet walking. Another of those three children had also come to our ER with a femur fracture, and we had reported it.

The county allowed that child to remain in the home. I am not privy to the details in any of these stories. I only know that three children died horribly, and that we saw two of them.

The advocate involved in the case that we didn't report told me she found solace in knowing that we did an assessment, consulted as a team, and made a judgment. We followed protocol, which in her eyes meant we didn't miss it.

In my eyes, not making the report was clearly a miss with fatal consequences. Yet, in the other case, we did make a report and the child still died. I can't know whether different actions on our part would have had different results, but I can't escape the profound sense of having failed both children.

$$\triangle$$

We don't always hear about our misses. I'm sure we had more. I know about one of mine. She was preschool age, maybe four. We'd just seen her for mild, nonspecific abdominal pain and discharged her with no abnormal findings. But she returned a half an hour later, curled up in agony. Her family had gone from the ER to a fast-food place across the street to get some lunch. She was feeling better and had a little food, but then collapsed, so they rushed her back.

The triage nurse ran back with the limp child in her arms, the charge nurse yelled out a room number, and staff flew out of all sides of the department to jump into action. In the room, I stood by her parents as the doctor shouted questions over the chaos, scrambling to piece together what happened. After additional tests she was diagnosed with injury to her spleen with no known mechanism. She was transferred by ambulance to a children's hospital in Augusta.

The next day our director told me she'd received a call from the ER director at the children's hospital asking why we didn't do a child abuse report. I was stunned. I missed it—me, who taught the class on recognizing abuse. I don't know whether the other hospital knew for sure that her injury was related to abuse, but they knew that a severe injury with no known accident history, especially in a young child, means you file a report.

Everything in the child's presentation led me to assume it was a purely medical ailment, not an inflicted injury, and no medical provider in our ER had implied otherwise. Advocates often catch the most obvious medical abuse injuries, like fractures, burns, and wounds, but we depend on physicians to tell us when a medical finding doesn't fit with the story we've been told. In the intensity of the moment, however, the doctor's focus is rightly on assessment and treatment—interventions to keep the child alive. It's the advocate who should be able to step back and ensure the pieces fit, or at least ask the doctor, *"How would this type of injury happen?"*

We had, of course, considered her parents "appropriate," a term I learned to hate. In the training classes I continued to do for new staff, I stressed the need for objectivity. Whether or not the parents seemed appropriately attached and dismayed by their child's suffering, certain injuries in very young children (head injuries, fractured femurs, abdominal injuries) should almost always be reported unless there is a known mechanism of injury, like a car accident.

During this time, we saw state protective services change their protocol. County workers were directed to follow up more quickly for younger children and intervene more significantly when the risk warranted it. I began telling these stories in the training classes—real examples of terrible mistakes, our sins of omission.

When a child came in with a suspicious injury, I encouraged advocates to ask themselves, "If the worst thing is true, if this is an inflicted injury, how much risk is this child in?"

A bruise from a parent's slap may seem equal to a small burn, but for a burn to have a shape, like of a cigarette butt, or a line of demarcation, requires a child to be held still, indicating more intent than a momentary flash of anger.

Of course, not all abuse leaves a mark. Emotional abuse is said to leave the deepest impact. It is present with all kinds of abuse but can also exist on its own. On average, we made one report each year based purely on observing emotional abuse—a parent's hostile, damaging verbal attacks that persisted during a visit, despite our attempts to stop them.

If a parent is continuously yelling, belittling, or shaming a child, we can try to distract the parent or support the child, but the most effective response is to empathize with the parent—being in the ER is stressful. We see people at their worst, but we must be at our best.

Supporting the parent does not mean we condone the parent's behavior, but we sympathize with the stress of the visit and acknowledge the concern they have for their child. We offer them coffee, a snack, or a toy for their child, or we give them a break and hold their child for a few minutes. If the verbal onslaught continues, we intercede more forcibly and report if needed.

△

A suspicious injury means a child may be at risk of further abuse. The same can be said of neglect, which is much more common but usually carries a lower risk. Injuries raise red flags, but neglect is all shades of gray.

As a social work student, I learned about the "good enough parent," the parent who is attached to their child and supplies them with the basics.[1] The good enough parent isn't perfect but doesn't need to be reported.

The danger of social workers projecting personal standards onto others' parenting styles is constant and not completely avoidable. Often neglect is a result of limited resources or education: The parent didn't realize the need to start the antibiotic right away; medical follow-up didn't happen because the clinic was closed the only time the parent was off work.

During my time in the ER, child protective services created a new program to support families that were reported and assessed to mostly

---

1. D. W. Winnicott, *Playing and Reality* (Tavistock Publications, 1971).

be in need of resources. Those reports were diverted to an outreach program to coordinate services, like signing up for Medicaid coverage, obtaining transportation, or finding a pediatrician.

As always in the ER, time was an obstacle—not reporting our "reasonable concerns" was a risk we couldn't take. We couldn't always know whether a report was merited. I'm sure this led to us over-reporting, which can damage the family and the very child we are trying to protect.

I took that potential damage seriously. In my journal, I noted a case (though I didn't include the child's age or injury) in which I was haunted by a child's expression when she was told she would be separated from her parents:

> *I sat in on the authorities' interview with the parents. When the parents told the child she couldn't go home with them, her face contorted in an agony of fear and sadness. I sat on my tears. Later, I tried to find some comfort that this child was attached to her parents, and they seemed attached to her. Maybe whatever went wrong can be fixed, healed, or understood. Seeing a hurt child with loving parents who are trying, full of remorse at failing, is painful. But seeing a child hurt without that caring parent—that is the thing that fills you with despair.*
>
> *I think about that toddler and how I hope she can go back home if that's a safe place. But always, as with any case that sticks with me, there is the critical self-review: sins of commission and omission. To the parents I said: "I know this has been an ordeal and that it continues. But you did the right thing to bring her in. She needed to be seen. It's clear that you love her and I'm hoping it works out for you and her."*

I didn't want the parents to regret bringing their child in, but surely they did. I didn't want to add to their hardships, but surely I did.

There is so much pain in this equation. And we are all flawed except the child.

In the class I taught, I used a DVD that featured a nurse who led education programs at her hospital. She spoke about the need to find empathy for the parents in these situations. This not only helps you work with the parents, but also opens your eyes to potential abuse or risk, because you realize that you are not looking for a monster. The nurse said that most working in emergency services recognize that we all have our own flaws and shortcomings, and that, as the saying goes, "There but for the grace of God go I."

Sins of Commission

I worried more about errors of omission than errors of commission because I believed I was more likely to miss something than to act in a way that would cause harm. Errors of commission are most likely to occur when you work outside of the policies of your organization, state law, or the ethics of your profession.

I often consulted guidelines, policy manuals, and our risk managers when I encountered new predicaments. But no source can cover everything. The balance between patients' rights and the law can be ambiguous and counter to what you feel is morally right.

When you go beyond the boundaries of your area of expertise or add extraneous information to what medical staff asked you to convey, you risk informational errors. This also happens when you move too quickly.

△

A "Doe" is a patient we cannot identify—John or Jane Doe is the typical designation. Quick identification is key for a patient's safety: We need a name and date of birth to find older records and to learn of allergies, medical issues, and the next of kin. An unidentified patient is at risk for being confused with another John or Jane Doe, and if a Doe chart doesn't get matched with the accurate name, the record of this visit may not get linked to their other records.

We started using a color-coding system for Doe patients in the aughts. This randomly assigns a color to a patient when we cannot quickly identify them. The colors in the system are vintage Crayola: saffron, meadow, sage, cerulean, fawn, and have no correlation to anything, including age, gender, race, or medical condition.

Patients have one medical history number and an account number for each individual visit. We must have an account number to order tests. The color name gives us that account number.

When an ambulance comes in with an unresponsive patient, even nonmedical staff flies into action. If the paramedics don't have the patient's name, advocates want to know whether anyone who knew them was on the scene. We alert the information desk that we have a Doe patient and instruct them to notify us of incoming visitors or calls.

If we're lucky, the paramedics walk in and hand us an ID card. Sometimes police roll in and provide the identification. More often, if the patient is coming from a car accident, police keep the ID card with them at the scene. This means we must find the officers to get the info. We don't delay care—the patient gets what they need as they need it— but we want a name as soon as possible.

As nurses swarm around the gurney, vying for position to start IV lines, an advocate becomes a pickpocket. The patient may still be wearing their pants when we thrust our hands deep inside the pockets, pulling out receipts, weapons, drugs. We scoop up the freshly cut clothes from the floor and retreat to a corner to rummage through them. We put the clothing scraps and shoes in a bag or a pile. Security witnesses our documentation of any money or credit cards, and together we seal it and send it to a lockbox. Then the advocate takes the wallet, purse, or phone to their desk to continue the hunt for the patient's identity and loved ones.

It is an odd thing to hold these fragments of someone's life. We become archivist detectives, sorting through cherished photos and random slips of paper in search of leads. A check with a phone number printed on it, a realtor's business card—everything is a potential clue. Patient confidentiality can be compromised in these cases because patient identification is part of medical safety.

We try to contact only the closest next of kin. But if the patient is unable to tell us who they are, we work on the assumptions that they want certain efforts made on their behalf. In considering whether I should violate the patient's privacy, I asked myself what I would want as that patient. I also asked myself what I would say to administrators or lawyers if accused of violating confidentiality. Could I defend my actions?

Sitting at my desk, sifting through the contents of a patient's pockets, knowing this person is fighting for their life and might be dying at that moment, I was desperate to find the people who loved them most, who wanted to be there at their side. This was my Level 1 of the triage system. Almost nothing was more important.

In addition to wanting the best care you can get as quickly as possible, most of us want our family alerted and with us right away. An entire team was working on the medical interventions, but I worked alone to find family. I might enlist another advocate or staff person, or I might get the police to help me, but it all started with me looking at the contents of those pockets to make connections.

Back before cell phones, I worried about my own pockets. Would they yield any clues about how to reach my husband?

△

My husband and I have different last names. We married in 1986, a time when not taking your husband's surname was unusual, at least in the South. When I encountered confusion about this—especially when people knew us separately and never put us together—I imagined the wheels in their mind spinning wildly. I'd say, "Yes, I'm one of *those* women," to help them reach the conclusion they seemingly couldn't conceive.

One of those women. Women who hope that holding on to their name will keep them from disappearing into their marriage, who are willing to risk awkwardness, confusion, and, in some places, even scorn.

According to the developmental psychologist Erik Erikson, I was in the Intimacy vs. Isolation stage when I made this decision. Erikson says that the challenge of this stage is to have a firm enough identity for yourself that you can "fuse" to another's identity "without fear you're going to lose something."[1] I wonder if Erikson ever had to do any fusing of his own.

Was keeping my name a crutch or an anchor? Did it divert me from the goal of this stage or help me achieve it? I had given up my name before, in a marriage that was fused to the point of enmeshment. That level of fusion didn't serve any of us—him, me, or the marriage. When I got my name back after the divorce, I swore I'd never give it up again. Now, with over thirty-five happy years in this marriage, I can say the choice to keep my name was an anchor. Feeling grounded in my identity, I was able to attach more deeply, to sustain real marital intimacy.

Choosing to not change your name when you marry probably seems like an inconsequential thing now, but back then, in small-town Georgia, it made a statement—a personal declaration I made and am proud of. But I wasn't very confident in the beginning. I said I would use my maiden name professionally and my married name socially. Some of *those kinds of women* did this then, to minimize offense, to give our mothers a way to soften the opinions of their friends, so their daughters didn't look so radical, so strident.

But it was too much to ask of myself, to carry around a second last name just because of what other people might think, other people that I mostly didn't care about. We gave our kids my husband's last name. I was told that this would be a problem: "People will assume they're not your kids."

I replied that anyone who mattered in our lives would know in two minutes that these were my kids. I had zero insecurities about my identity as their mother. I'd seen how adoptive parents reach past genetics to find not just a tether to their hearts, but also a rock-hard place in their guts, radiating a fierce claim to parenthood and to their children.

But I had not yet started working in the ER when I made my decision about names for myself and my children. I did not know that there are times when you don't want there to be two minutes before

---

1. Erik Erikson, *Childhood and Society* (W. W. Norton & Company, 1993), 263.

someone links you to those you love most. I could ensure that my info
was on every form for my kids, and that their friends' parents knew
all our names and numbers, but if someone had my pocket and purse
contents at their desk, could they link me to *them*?

If I was in a car accident, paramedics in town might recognize me,
but identification was more likely if I was brought to "my" hospital. I
taped a scrap of paper on the back of my driver's license with my hospital of choice and my husband's name and number. I kept my license
this way for years, until I had a cell phone with my emergency contacts.

Of course, none of that is any good if your phone is locked; thus
cell phones often do not give a quick solution to the problem of identification. Ensure your phone has an emergency option that leads to
a Medical ID (red asterisk) on the home screen. This leads to a list of
emergency contacts that can be accessed even if your phone is locked.

Perhaps you think it's more likely that your phone would be stolen
and this information misused than that you'd be in an accident. I can't
speak to the statistics of those probabilities, just to my experience,
which is admittedly warped: I've stared helplessly at a locked screen
while the patient is alone and those who love them remain unaware.

Besides the risk of not being connected to your family, there is the
danger of someone making the wrong connection—accurate identification depends on accurate information. If you keep your phone locked
with no emergency access, if you carry the wrong ID, the wrong family
could be notified. This may seem like the most far-fetched improbability, but remember in the realm of worst-case scenarios, anything can
and does happen. And it happened to me.

△

My rush started around four that morning, when the phone woke me
up. It was the advocate who was supposed to leave at three, calling me
in. She had stayed late with a death, and now that she was about to
walk out the door, three DOA patients came in, two boys and a girl,
college-aged, from the scene of a car crash.

In those days we were on call from three to seven a.m., the only hours during which no advocate was scheduled to be in the ER. Everyone had their preference for which night they chose to take call. I took call on the nights before I was scheduled to come in at seven a.m., preferring to think of being called in as just starting my day a few hours early. That way, call never interfered with my day-off plans, though it did make an already hard workday much harder.

Before going to bed the night before, I'd pack my lunch, set my clothes out, and put the phone by my bed. ER policy states that when you are called in, you must arrive to clock in within thirty minutes. Once your phone rang, that clock was punched and running, and you were hurled into a game of Beat the Clock with the worst prizes ever.

"Winning" meant you got to take over the emotional and logistical issues of some horrible situation while you were barely awake, but winning also meant that you avoided a violation of policy. These violations were tracked and counted; accrue a few and you would be fired. As soon as the call woke me, my adrenaline surged, and I sprang out of bed.

The advocate I relieved stayed to give me the report. The death that she had worked earlier was also a young person from a crash. He'd come in hours earlier and died on our gurney. His family was still there, clustered in and around the patient's room, sobbing, holding each other. His was one of those deaths that touched staff deeply. Those that worked at his bedside now cried in the nurses' station, with the advocate comforting them.

It was eerie to walk into this aftermath, like coming into a war zone after a bomb went off. The ER was in ruins, and I was an outsider who stumbled in knowing nothing about their experience. I had caught the ER in a rare pause, licking its wounds. In a moment, it would reset and resume business as usual. But none of this had anything to do with why I was called in.

Except for the grieving in and around trauma room two, the ER was mostly empty. A room on the nonurgent side, around the corner from the trauma bays, was closed for patients because it held three gurneys with three bodies in bags. The advocate said she felt bad for neglecting them, but all her energy went to caring for the family of the patient who had arrived alive. There was nothing medical to be done for these three; they had been pronounced dead at the scene.

Usually, the advocate would have worked on ID'ing them and contacting family. She was known for often staying late, for being reluctant to utilize her coworker on call, preferring to finish cases herself. But she was now over an hour past the end of her shift and knew the work with the DOAs was going to be a lengthy process not suited to a handoff.

Identifying a patient and finding their family is like a maze. Many routes will lead you to the treasure in the center—in this case, the patient's name and the phone number of someone who knows them—but choices must be made each step of the way: which turn to take, which lead to follow. Choosing a way in, a direction to start, was the hardest decision and would have the most impact on how long the process would take. Sometimes you can't crack the puzzle before the end of your shift and must hand it over, but taking someone's place in a maze means either trying to follow their way-finding logic or tossing their logic out and starting over with your own. This puzzle was untouched, waiting for me to solve it.

$$\triangle$$

The three DOA patients were also made Doe patients—though we had their driver's licenses. Because no medical treatment was needed, there had not been the usual rush to verify their identification or assign one.

A call to the college police confirmed they were not students at the university in our town. Presumably they were visiting friends who were students here, but we had no idea who those friends were. Facebook did not yet exist.

I contacted State Patrol. They had the info from the driver's licenses and verified the names and family contacts. They had not contacted any of the families and did not seem inclined to do that anytime soon. They were the night shift, and ready to punt that task to their day shift relief and go home.

No one wants to contact the families. When the ER is functioning simply as a holding area—a place to pronounce the patient, verify identity, and complete the required paperwork before transporting them to the morgue in the hospital's basement—it can be argued that contacting family is not our responsibility. Notification could be deferred to the police or to the coroner. In my experience, it can be hours before that contact is made. I was also concerned about how the families would be informed by those authorities and what support they would receive.

Where the body goes, the family often follows. Families came to the ER even if we provided no medical care. Sometimes the police would tell the families that their loved one had been in an accident and they should go to the ER. Families rushed to our door, believing their loved one was still alive, desperate to see them. The police may have felt we were the safest place for families to hear the worst news, whereas I thought it was better for families to get this news at home.

Having the bodies meant we would deal with the aftermath of the notification process. If I was going to be involved with the families, I preferred to be involved in the notification. Those families felt like our responsibility, my responsibility.

In later years, as our ER got busier, DOA patients didn't even stop in the ER. They went straight to the morgue. The coroners notified families. Advocates were involved only when family requested to go to the morgue or needed resources. Most often the family would go directly to the funeral home and skip the ER altogether.

This seems better for everyone: It frees up the advocate to work with patients receiving medical care, it keeps our treatment rooms open for patients instead of serving as a family visitation area, and families bypass the harsh environment of the ER.

But in those earlier days, if the charge nurse felt we had a room to spare, it was considered a courtesy to keep a deceased patient in the ER for a short while so the family didn't have to view their loved one in the morgue. In the ER, families saw their loved one in a private room with lights as soft as we could make them. Cushy chairs were pulled up to the bedside and a full box of Kleenex placed on the table. Whereas the morgue required a long walk to the basement, where we'd pull out a metal gurney from a refrigerated walk-in, with the patient zipped up in a body bag.

△

Unlike the coroner or State Patrol, who were usually handling multiple issues, I could devote myself to the three Doe patients. The addresses I was given were all out of town, two in metro-Atlanta, where almost everyone has a troublesome commute to work. It was a weekday morning, so those parents would be leaving their homes soon, and home landlines were the only numbers I had. They would be unreachable all day if I didn't call them now.

It might have been possible to find those parents at work, but that was uncertain, and would take more time. Also, delivering this message to someone at work seemed like a sucker punch—knocking them to their knees while they are out in the world, surrounded by people they may not know, having to figure out how to tell their spouse the impossible as they drive home. Being careful about how we tell the worst news is not just an act of compassion; we want to protect the family's safety as much as possible.

No one is in a hurry for bad news, but news about your child should never be delayed. I was determined to reach the families before they left their homes. It was now after five a.m. I had to act quickly. The parents lived between one to three hours away. In each case it was the father who answered the phone.

I said who I was, and that I worked in the *emergency room*, saying the full phrase instead of "ER." I said it slowly and then stopped. I let it sink in, hating that my words made their stomachs drop, that I couldn't negate the seriousness of the moment by rushing into reassurance that their child was OK, or at least alive.

I confirmed the father's name, confirmed the name of his child, and then spoke the words that stalk every parent's nightmare: "I'm so sorry, but I have terrible news . . ."

I reached them all while they were at home. None of them chose to come to the ER; I sent their children to the morgue. The treatment room they shared was emptied, and a living patient needing care was brought into it.

Another advocate came in for his shift and covered all of the ER as I worked at a desk in the nurses' station, completing three sets of paperwork and phone calls to the coroner and the organ donation agency.

Somewhere three families were huddled in a fog of devastation, making decisions no one ever prepared them for. One by one, they called me back, all the dads, with the names of the funeral homes.

One by one, their children were picked up from the morgue by those funeral homes. It was now afternoon; I'd been on shift about ten hours. The last one picked up was the girl. I knew because Security was being careful, calling me to double-check before they released the body, even though the name of the funeral home that came for her matched the one I'd written on the form. They didn't want the wrong body to go to the wrong place.

The day shift charge nurse was a friend. Diane was all kinds of smart: flow-smart, masterfully managing room assignments, the arrival and discharge of patients, and allocation of staff; medical-smart, a damn good nurse who kept her skills sharp; people-smart, skillfully handling staff, doctors, administration, and any random problem that reached her. Now she walked up to me, holding her cordless phone, her eyes wide.

Diane asked the caller to wait a moment and she put her hand over the receiver. She was speaking to the girl who died. Someone had seen her on campus with the friend she was visiting and told her, sputtering, that she was dead.

Listening to the phone, Diane narrowed her eyes in a look to me that said she was hearing an excuse she didn't buy. Her face said "incoming bullshit," but her voice remained professional as she repeated the words—the words of the not-dead girl telling Diane she had lost her driver's license recently. The girl on the phone implied that this other girl, the one who died, had apparently "found" her license. My world froze. Diane waited. It was my move.

"Apologize to her and explain, then call PR and Risk Management. I'm calling the funeral home to bring her back." The not-dead girl had called her parents straightaway, so I didn't have to call them back. After reaching the funeral home, I alerted Security to be ready to reopen the morgue.

Word spread among the college students. One called to give us the likely name of the girl who had died. She was under twenty-one. The driver's license we found on her belonged to her friend who was old enough to drink—the girl Diane spoke with, the one missing her license.

There was no time to give in to the shame and horror of what I'd done. I still had a body to identify and a family to notify. I made another call to another father, home from his day at work. I told him what happened and that I believed this was his daughter, but we had to be sure. He didn't ask to come; I insisted. I would not risk a further mistake. Never again did I assume someone was who we thought they were until someone who knew them came and saw them.

When the father arrived, I met him in the Family Room, and I called Security to meet us in the basement to unlock the morgue. On TV, you see morgue identification all the time, but in our ER, it didn't happen often. The dad was steady enough to take the stairs, a shortcut out the back of the ER through the ambulance bay, facing west into the setting sun. For fourteen hours I'd been inside this horror. But it was nothing compared to the horror of your child lying in a morgue.

Security met us at the unmarked door. Years later an advocate would create a warmer space for family inside this viewing room, with chairs and a lamp, the walls painted a soft beige, with one of those mass-produced prints of a landscape painting—a meadow or maybe a river—hanging on the wall. A curtain would be added in front of the large industrial refrigerator door. Going in alone, we would roll the body out and pull the curtain shut, before bringing family in, hiding the cruelty of the obvious.

On this evening I worked with what I had. While Security stood in the gray hall a few feet from the dad, knowing to give him some space, to bear the awkward silence rather than attempt small talk, I prepared the viewing room. I switched on the harsh fluorescent light, which revealed chips and dings in the unfortunate dusty-rose wall paint, evidence of maneuvering collisions in the tight space. I tugged the heavy refrigerator door open and walked into the dark case, careful to brace the door to keep it from closing while I was inside. It wouldn't have locked me in, but if it shut, I'd be in the cold dark with the deceased.

I pulled the gurney out of the refrigerator and into the viewing area. I unzipped the body bag and covered it with one of the soft cotton blankets kept stocked there just for this purpose. The blanket, like the curtain that came later, is a tool of subtle deception—as if the starkness of death's cold reality can be assuaged by fabric. The box of tissues in place on the wobbly stained table, I opened the door and brought the dad in.

It was his daughter. He didn't hesitate; he didn't cry. He gave me the funeral home name. It was dusk now as we went back up the stairs. I walked him to his car. He said he was OK to drive. I gave him my name, the ER number, and my condolences.

Back at the nurses' station, the night shift workers were coming in. I finished the new set of paperwork, made all the calls, and drove home in the dark to my children.

I'd let my husband know I'd be late because it was a "bad day." If he told our kids anything, it would be just that. We had dinner and did all the bedtime routines. I hugged my children tight. Once they were in bed, the two of us sat on the couch and talked about what happened. I needed his help with this one, someone to tell me it wasn't my fault, which of course he did emphatically. I really wanted to believe him.

$$\triangle$$

I was off the next day and wanted to stay home and hide in my bed. But plans had been made to meet my parents at an art exhibit in Atlanta. They were traveling two hours to get there, and we already had our tickets. Part of me was glad to get out of town, envisioning the story blowing up behind me in my hospital and town.

I didn't say anything to my parents about what had happened. By then I was an expert at compartmentalization, leaving my work at work. Or so I thought. My life outside the ER often felt like walking through someone else's movie—an external world that didn't match my internal reality. My insides burbled with images, sensations, and feelings I would not release, unwilling to contaminate this serene outside world. I strolled through the exhibit as if I appreciated the priceless art around us, making remarks to my parents.

My parents. Their daughter still alive . . . years they had with me, seeing me graduate college, get married, have children . . . my children, my husband, alive at home. Three families in three other homes consumed in a nightmare and a fourth injured needlessly at my hand. How was today for those families?

That fourth family was angry. They called hospital administration with their outrage: Why would I assume it was their daughter just because their daughter's driver's license was on the patient? Their daughter simply lost her license. People lose their license all the time.

I don't know if anyone told them that it was quite a coincidence that their daughter's license had been "found" by a friend of hers, a friend who happened to resemble her, a friend who was under drinking age in a town known for college parties.

Most likely this wasn't said outright unless the parents persisted. The administrators were parents too. We all knew that if that wave of paralyzing fear came to our door and knocked us to our knees, we would seek firmer ground—a way to believe it would never happen again. We would want to reclaim our absolutism, our belief that our child was always going to be safe. We had taken that from them—*I'd* taken that from them. And they wanted me punished. But I was defended by hospital administration, my actions and intentions explained, and my remorse alluded to.

Diane told me that a fellow advocate was openly critical of me when other staff were talking about the incident and expressed their support. She picked apart my decisions, explaining how she could never make that mistake. Diane said that the staff had shut down that advocate, refusing to let her words go unchallenged. I felt I deserved her blame, but it was comforting to know the team had protectively closed ranks around me. Many remarked that those fourth parents should "just be grateful for the life of their child." But it's unlikely for anyone drenched in that kind of fear to see it as a gift. Anger feels safer than fear. Almost anyone who can swap fear for anger will do so, myself included.

The complaints from the family dwindled, and the chatter among staff moved on to the next thing. And I was left with a story that I wished I could bury. Instead, I shared it with advocates in training in hopes of preventing a similar mistake by them, for the next patient and for the next family.

Acknowledging it here doesn't purge the pain. I tried to talk myself out of including it. There are many stories I will not tell—why tell this one? In these pages I scrutinize so many aspects of the system and the people in it; I can't justify ducking one of my worst failures. It shaped me, as failures tend to do.

I know how it feels to commit an error of devastating impact, an error that may have been avoided if I had not taken a wrong turn in that maze of decisions. I didn't intend to cause needless pain; I thought acting quickly was acting compassionately. But after that day, I took pauses between my turns in the maze. I moved a little more slowly, became more humble, less confident, less judgmental, and more forgiving.

Losing the War Against Reality

I used to scoff at the term *burnout*. I thought I knew what burnout looked like: calling in sick when you weren't or because the job made you sick, or, when you did make it to work, hardly working. I thought burnout meant you no longer cared about those you served or the organization you worked for. None of that was ever true for me.

An academic paper I read defined *burnout* as "prolonged response to chronic emotional and interpersonal stressors on the job, determined by the dimensions of exhaustion, cynicism, and inefficacy."[1] *Inefficacy* meaning without the power or capacity to produce the effect desired. Check. Perhaps burnout wasn't just a personal failing.

But *secondary traumatic stress* sounded more noble. Having burnout was a character flaw, but having secondary traumatic stress gave you a halo. The person suffering with secondary traumatic stress (STS) did not directly experience the trauma, but they took care of the person who did. The symptoms of STS resemble the symptoms experienced by those who suffer with PTSD, post-traumatic stress disorder.[2]

To measure STS, a tool was created called the Secondary Traumatic Stress Scale.[3] In 2013, having worked in the ER for twenty-two years,

---

1. Christina Maslach, Wilmar B. Schaufeli, and Michael P. Leiter, "Job Burnout," *Annual Review of Psychology*, 52 (2001): 397–422.
2. American Psychiatric Association. *Desk Reference to the Diagnostic Criteria from DSM-5*, (American Psychiatric Publishing, 2013).
3. Brian E. Bride, Margaret R. Robinson, Bonnie Yegidis, and Charles R. Figley, "Development and Validation of the Secondary Traumatic Stress Scale," *Research on Social Work Practice*, 14 (2004): 27–35. The test is at: https://theacademy.sdsu.edu/wp-content/uploads/2019/09/STSSwithscoreinterpretation.pdf.

I attended a presentation on STS. Attendees took the survey to see where we fell on the scale. Each of the seventeen items on the scale was a statement, for example, *I thought about my work with clients when I didn't want to.* This alludes to the presence of intrusive thoughts.

Each statement has five possible responses, ranging from "never" (which is assigned zero points) to "very often" (which is assigned five points). After responding to all of the statements, you add up the points for each of your answers to get your total score. A total score below 28 indicates little or no STS; 28–37 indicates mild STS; 38–43 is moderate; 44–48 is high; 49 and above is severe.

My score was 54. I was surprised. Among my fives and fours there were also threes and twos. Isn't this what normal looks like? At least, "normal" for working in the realm of worst-case scenarios? I didn't feel "severe." I didn't want a halo stained with pathology! I was *fine.*

The term *compassion fatigue* was coined in 1992 by a nurse named Carla Joinson as a less stigmatizing label than secondary traumatic stress.[4] Some people use the terms interchangeably; some researchers define compassion fatigue as a combination of burnout and STS.[5]

Does it really matter whether it's burnout, STS, or compassion fatigue? Only if you want to get better. STS indicates the issue is the work itself, burnout points the finger at the organization you're working for, and compassion fatigue can be a combination of both.

Some of the self-care recommendations, like tending to your health, prioritizing relationships that nurture you, connecting to a hobby or community project unrelated to work, or spending time in nature, are beneficial strategies for any of the three. But if the issue is more organizational—powerlessness in dealing with structural inequities, or a lack of autonomy in changing what directly impacts your work (the pace, hours, processes, salary, or amount of support and appreciation)—self-care remedies can only go so far. I tried them all anyway.

---

4. Carla Joinson, "Coping with Compassion Fatigue," *Nursing* 22, no. 4 (1992): 116, 118–120.
5. J. Eric Gentry, Anna B. Baranowsky, and Kathleen Dunning, "The Accelerated Recovery Program (ARP) for Compassion Fatigue," in *Treating Compassion Fatigue,* ed. Charles R. Figley (Brunner-Routledge, 2002), 123–137.

△

My first favorite cure was tennis. I came from a tennis family, my dad and brother always among the best players anywhere we lived. I was taught to play at an early age but didn't want to compete with their reputations. My mother advocated for me to get a horse—my biggest childhood salvation until I met my best friend at age thirteen.

Mom enjoyed horseback riding and gave my brother and me lessons. The idea was that I would provide the essential regular care for this family pet that everyone would ride. A couple of times a year someone else rode, but only with my help. Each day I pedaled my bike a few miles to the stable to groom, feed, and ride, and to muck out the stall. I was nine years old. I loved it.

It was incredible to be in charge of this wondrous, huge beast, said to be part draft horse. The responsibility and the freedom of having hours each day to myself to do this job however I wanted to were thrilling. Having a horse gave me membership in a gang of stable girls, some friendly, some frightening, all more interested in their animals than in each other. Most of us were misfits. Traditional codes of behavior didn't apply at the barn—I learned how to curse and smoke, break minor laws, and ride backward. When we moved, we sold that horse, but soon bought another who I kept until I was fifteen.

I joined my family on the courts often enough to develop and maintain some skills, and in high school I joined the tennis team. I wasn't a star like my brother, but the girls' team was small and prone to losing. Showing up was good enough.

After high school, I didn't play tennis for years. My husband was an occasional player, so we took intermediate-level lessons as a couple. This was supposed to be a new activity for us to do together, but when the lessons ended, only a women's team needed members. I joined it.

I had dismissed women tennis players as conventional country club types, but this team was more like the girls at the stable. They played with gusto and laughter, never taking themselves, each other, or the match too seriously. They were career women with diverse interests and perspectives that meshed with mine. Suddenly my life was infused with a vitality and hilarity that rivaled the ER's intensity.

I played with them for over six years and had the most outrageous fun of my life, a joyful distraction from work. Sometimes the needs of the ER would interfere with playing, and a teammate joked that I needed to get my priorities straight: "You gotta quit that damn job." I loved the idea, but I would not quit the damn job for years and years.

I did quit playing tennis, though. When I got tendonitis in one arm, I kept playing. When it got worse, I sat out of matches but didn't change anything else in my life. My other arm got tendonitis. They didn't heal until I finally quit using them as much as possible. No tennis and no exercise except walking or riding a stationary bike, hands free.

I looked fit and was embarrassed to ask for help. At the grocery store, I asked them to pack the bags light. When even that hurt, I swallowed my pride and asked them to carry the bags to the car, explaining my arms didn't work. At home, the kids brought the bags in. I limited typing at work and quit writing for pleasure. I wore splints on my arms, and they hurt every day. I assumed this was my new normal.

I thought of the patients we see in the ER who live with daily pain, and how I never thought that would be me. This was not a debilitating ailment, and the pain was not all-consuming, but it was persistent. It was a year before my arms quit hurting all the time.

My life grew back, and eventually I could take feeling good for granted. But I wasn't willing to risk injury again by resuming tennis. Besides, my team was no longer intact. Thankfully the friendships remain.

During that year of arm rest, I looked for another consuming distraction and found local film projects. Acting was what I knew best from high school and college. I got cast in a few roles but found more enjoyment in production. Being a larger part of shaping the project was gratifying. Films became my next favorite antidote to the stress of the ER.

My most exciting film project was underway in the spring of 2007, when I was part of the production crew for a locally made independent feature film, *Pushin' Up Daisies*, directed by Patrick Franklin. Much of the filming was done on weekends and late nights to accommodate crew members, such as myself, who had other jobs, and the dozens of extras we needed to be zombies. As extras coordinator, I was head wrangler of that zombie horde. This was before *The Walking Dead* aired, but zombies were already popular, and we had no problem recruiting volunteers.

I had no interest in being a zombie, and my hands were full with communications and coordination, but when the stuntwoman cast for a featured zombie role (the mother of the main character) wasn't able to come, I found myself volunteering. For three days I put my clipboard and phone down and got into zombie makeup appropriate for a woman who'd been lying dead in a lake for a few years.

There was a house-haunting scene at night that required I be sprayed with cold water between each take to maintain my dripping wet countenance, but mostly I had to walk in a lopsided stride that never quite satisfied the director. Because I had never aspired to be a zombie, I had neglected to learn this critical skill. I hobbled up and down dirt roads all over the countryside, trying everyone's patience as each actor and crew member tried infusing my zombie walk with more reality.

The big scene came on the third day of filming, when my character returns to the place of her death—the lake. With a weight belt strapped on to aid me in sinking down in the water, I joined my "husband" (whose zombie walk elicited only praise). We returned to our watery deaths, slowly sinking down as we tottered into the lake. When the water covered our heads, I realized that the lake had a current. It swept me out deeper than expected, to where I couldn't touch. I'm a strong swimmer, but because of the weight belt, I couldn't keep my head up, and it never occurred to me to simply unbuckle the belt, as the safety coordinator had instructed. But fortunately, that safety guy saw my flailing hands and was a fast swimmer. As he made his way to me, the actor playing my husband was able to splash closer. He also couldn't touch but wasn't being drug down by the belt. I could have just been led to dry land, but safety guy put me in a rescue hold and swam me out. I was relieved but embarrassed. Thankfully, we got the shot.

Kinda almost drowning isn't the reason I quit working on films; rather, it was the kinda almost falling asleep at the wheel when driving home at three in the morning. In my mid-forties, I was too old for that work, especially with having a more than full-time job at which I saw what happened when people did fall asleep while driving.

Because I was late to indie filmmaking, I decided the best investment of my time was not on set but at my desk, writing. This was a giant uncomfortable step away from constant motion, from the attribute that defined this era of my life—Act. I'd been like a plate spinner, certain that if I twirled them fast enough, we'd all make it through unbroken.

I started writing scripts. Two short scripts I wrote were produced by local groups, and I was in the thick of those productions, contributing in any way that I could. Writing gave me control over content; I could dictate the story being told. A feature-length script of mine was optioned by an LA-based production company but ultimately never made, a fate befalling most optioned scripts. But writing was rewarding despite the outcome. According to Lewis Carroll, "Imagination is the only weapon in the war against reality." In my home, I could release my imagination from the compartment I now kept it in. Unfurling it at my desk, I didn't have to see or think about real life's daily menu of horrors.

I constructed worlds, starting with that of a young woman laid low by her father's death, stalked by predatory dreams. I followed with a comedy about a tennis team of misfits. I wrote a sci-fi script of a near future on Earth where a new implanted technology separates humans. There's a fairy tale about a princess who learns survival skills from the witch in the woods, and a horror comedy with squirrels making their bid for world domination. And, yes, there is a story about a social worker. Recovering from her work in child protective services, she works in guest relations for a hotel, hiding from her past and the case that went terribly wrong. But denial doesn't work for her either, and her happy ending comes only when she faces those ghosts of the past.

Clearly, they weren't all cheerful, fun stories, yet I commonly received the critical note that my stakes weren't high enough—I don't inflict enough suffering onto my characters. My worlds may contain worst-case scenarios, but the heroine always succeeds, and with less than the usual agony.

$$\triangle$$

ER nurses rank highest on the scale of secondary traumatic stress. They rank even higher than social workers in child protective services.[6] Among the medical staff I've encountered, from doctors to paramedics to nursing techs, there is a resistance to acknowledging the toll the work takes, and this can keep them from getting the help they need.

Peer support and debriefing sessions are often cited as helpful coping strategies, but given a choice to participate, staff usually chooses home, sleep, and family over giving more of their time and energy to a place that is making them stressed, anxious, frustrated, and exhausted. Building support into the structure of shifts, into the meetings we're required to attend, is a step in this direction. But sometimes a system is too stretched to even have meetings, and staff are too tired to check in with each other, their teammates.

More than the individual tasks and the issues inherent in the hospital, it was the overwhelming scope of the work itself that wore me down. No hospital can overcome the broken system that is health care in our country. Fractures in this system mean a relentless churn of patients. Traumas are one thing, but illnesses worsened by the absence of basic care or the complexity of addiction and mental health issues reflect the lack of a coordinated system, and there was almost no sign for hope of improvement.

But then came the Affordable Care Act, or Obamacare. I thought the system-wide change I had waited for all these years was finally here, or at least had begun. There was the possibility of medical insurance for so many who had never had it, which meant they could see primary care doctors and sometimes specialists. But because Georgia did not accept the monies for expanding Medicaid (due to politicians'

6. Bride, Robinson, Yegidis, and Figley, "Development and Validation of the Secondary Traumatic Stress Scale."

fears of appearing receptive to federal assistance), the potential benefit was not fully realized. From my view in the trenches, it was hard to perceive a significant positive impact. The population around our hospital grew, and rural hospitals around us closed. Our census climbed with no end in sight.

Sharon Salzberg, cofounder of the Insight Meditation Society and author of eleven books on well-being, prefers the term *empathy fatigue* to *compassion fatigue*. She believes that the word *compassion* implies boundaries and is distinct from empathy in that compassion avoids overidentification with the person or the cause you are focused on.[7]

Salzberg encourages us to continue to lean toward compassion as a tool for the long game—a way to connect to others and build the resilience needed to stay in the role of helper. I want to believe that, despite my emotional wounds, my compassion is still intact. I have those detachment skills; I can care without taking in the pain. Yet, there is a part of myself that sits in judgment, that thinks if I don't feel the pain of the person in front of me, I'm just phoning it in, going through the motions.

Yet I don't expect myself to feel everything with each person, and my helping a patient doesn't depend on experiencing their pain. In fact, helping from an emotional place complicates your ability to help—"helping getting in the way of *helping*." But when I do an internal scan and find no emotion resonating, I worry that I've lost my ability to connect. That my armor is so thick, nothing can get through.

In my fifties, as feelings of disconnection, generalized anxiety, and my inability to cry became routine, I began to fear that this work had changed me forever.

---

7. Sharon Salzberg, *Real Change: Mindfulness to Heal Ourselves and the World* (Flatiron Books, 2020), 128–131.

LISTEN

How to Stay Out of the ER

If you skipped to this part of the book, spoiler alert: I am not a medically trained professional. This list is not medical advice. When in doubt, go.

1. **Don't stick things into orifices that are not designed for those orifices.**
2. **Take your medicine regularly.** Problems doing that? Talk to your doctor. Don't have a doctor? You're not alone. Try: findahealthcenter.hrsa.gov. If your doctor often tells you to go to the ER, find another doctor.
3. **Don't drive when impaired.**
4. **Don't bike, Rollerblade, or skateboard when impaired.**
5. **Don't walk when impaired.**
6. **Don't get so impaired.**
7. **Living with weapons can lead to unintended injuries.**
8. **Living with physically or emotionally abusive people will cause distress and risks harm.** You deserve to be safe. Please let someone help you make a careful plan.
9. **Do all those things you're tired of hearing about:** Wear your seat belt; keep your car maintained; don't text while driving; know your allergies and take precautions; monitor chronic health problems closely, including mental health needs; eat well; wash your hands; don't smoke; move your body safely and unimpaired.

Or ignore this advice . . . and upgrade your underwear drawer.

10. **But seriously: *Come in as needed.*** There is nothing too weird, too small, or too stupid for an ER visit. No one is perfect, and we've seen it all—we will not be surprised.

11. **And relax . . .** Nothing is under control, but we will take care of you.

We Can Save Your Life—Do We Really Have to Be Nice?

"Is there anything else? I have the time." That sounds like something a front desk person at a boutique hotel would say. It was a phrase that one of the ER directors encouraged staff to use, especially the advocates, who never felt they had that time to offer but who were rightfully expected to lead customer service efforts.

This was in the late nineties, when expectations for customer service grew in the hospital industry. Patient satisfaction surveys were now required, and the data from those surveys shaped how hospitals were ranked and judged for accreditation. Such data would become public, posted on websites.

Hospitals found themselves taking tips from companies like famous amusement parks I can't name and well-known fast-food franchises—businesses known for excellent service but having nothing to do with health care. Hospitals also hired glitzy executives from the hospitality industry to give inspirational talks and hawk their books revealing the secrets of their success.

Good business is good business, and in the United States hospitals are a business. But hospitals are also staffed with people who feel called to work there, who are driven to make a difference in something deeper than customer experience or the CEO's profit margin.

There are commonalities in human expectations and behavior—companies who excel at customer service have strategies that can translate to other organizations. But ask an experienced ER nurse to read a book about how these companies specializing in vacations and food go the extra mile, and that nurse will conclude that you know nothing about their work and why they do it.

One tactic these nonmedical companies advocated was scripting—using specific phrases at specific times. There is a saying in ERs that the more upright a person is, the more they resemble a customer rather than a patient—patients with emergent and urgent conditions lie down, nonurgent patients sit up.

No one said we should script our response to critical patients and their families, though certainly there were things one should not say or even imply, like that the way they mourned was wrong—shushing them; responding to their wail of "This is my fault!" with "You shouldn't feel that way"; pushing a box of tissues into their hands, giving the unspoken direction to "clean up, get yourself under control."

Communication with a customer patient is far more complicated. The more stable they are, the more they notice details, like the impatient attitude of the registration clerk, the staff laughing loudly, or that their room is way too cold. Getting annoyed takes energy. I had very few complaints from patients who came to us in critical condition.

But there are points in an ER visit, times of transition, that function as opportunities, when the right kind of communication can help shape a perception. The wait to be seen is estimated as "within an hour," instead of "a few minutes"; negative test results mean "We didn't find anything," instead of "There's nothing wrong with you"; and putting off a request is "Sure, as soon as I can," instead of "No, I'm too busy" or "That's not my job." As we close the door to their treatment room we say, "We're closing this door to protect your privacy," instead of "We don't want you to hear us chatting in the nurses' station." We intentionally use that phrase "protect your privacy," which will be part of a question on their satisfaction survey: "Was your privacy protected?"

If we could clarify our process for the patients and families, they might have more realistic expectations, give us better rankings on the survey, and be less inclined to complain. They'd be happier, we'd be happier. We wouldn't be changing the care we give, just helping patients to recognize that care as excellent.

But ER staff did not want to spout lines that someone told them to say. They were doing authentic work; using a script felt fake. The more specific the direction was, the more vigorously the staff rebelled. But administration was adamant. The culture of "We're here to save your life, not bring you a warm cookie" would have to change.

Changing ER culture meant confronting the culture of the past. Our seasoned staff came on board in an era when they expected to be judged by their skills. As we rolled into this new customer service era, they were handed the books, required to attend presentations, and coached, but no one really expected longtime staff to embrace the new warm and fuzzy ER. Fundamental change would come through young hires who could be molded. New employees in all positions, medical to clerical, attended orientation sessions with a focus on customer service.

Directors reinforced their support for these values by integrating customer service data and techniques into staff meetings, reading aloud letters of compliments and complaints—making customer service a respected element of good medical care. It fell to middle managers to work with individual staff to break down the feedback into "teachable moments."

One of my directors made it personal: She told staff that she wanted an ER that she could send her family to and be confident that they would get good care. She explained that "good care" included being treated with respect and compassion *from the perspective of the patient and family.*

Perception matters. In my world, perception mattered almost as much as facts. Facts frame the border of an incident, but perception fills in the picture with impressions, colors, and tone. Communication was often a major part of the patient's or family members' issue when we failed to clarify why we were doing what we were doing. Communication in the moment can change perceptions.

△

Soon after customer service ratings became public, the national accreditation organization added a requirement for hospitals to create and maintain a grievance response system. That system had to include documentation, administrative involvement as indicated, follow-ups with employees if needed, and contact with the person making the complaint. This level of response is time-consuming. If I handled grievances, the director and ER nurse managers could focus on running the department.

At this point we had already resolved the primary source of complaints—our visitor policy. The old policy required a doctor's permission to allow a visitor to join a patient in a treatment room. If family rode in on the ambulance with the patient, an advocate was asked to separate them from the patient and take them to the waiting room. Pro-family nurses didn't wait for permission and simply brought the family back themselves. Nurses reluctant to defy a physician played by the rules, leaving the family to stew in their worries and frustration, with the patient alone in the room, ultimately requiring the advocate to ask for the doctor's permission.

We changed that visitor policy through a multidisciplinary group of ER staff, including a physician, with the goal of making our policy more visitor friendly. The committee kept returning to one question: What would you want if the patient were your family, or if you were the patient? The policy we created did not routinely separate family from patients, and even created a process to allow visitation during a code, a way for family to be in the room when their loved one died.

Advocates had to limit the number of family members who could be present during a code. We had to prepare them and stay beside them. We couldn't always get them to the bedside; they might stand in the back of the room as staff did compressions.

To *call a code* means to end it, to halt the efforts to resuscitate the patient. The time of death is whatever time the code is called. When family was in the room, a strange thing often happened: Family started calling the code, telling us to stop. They could see the futility of continuing and the violence of the attempt. They might not be ready to let their loved one go, but they did anyway—out of compassion.

As my work shifted to more follow-up care and complaint

management, I reduced the time I spent in direct patient care. Eventually, I had no assigned shifts but worked in the ER as needed when we had gaps in coverage. Mostly, I worked behind the curtain in the administrative post-visit world. This was my new playing field, where I got to try to make a difference on the back end.

This took me away from the frequent stress of seeing trauma raw, the patient straight from the scene, the shock descending on families as they got the news of their nightmares, often from me.

My years-long routine of leaving my house by 6:20, driving with a slice of cheese toast in my lap and my first cup of coffee in hand— forcing myself to eat and drink before I arrived, knowing I may not eat or drink for hours—gave way to a more easeful existence. I had some control over my hours and an office with easy access to good coffee and a mini fridge. Work was almost civilized.

The stress was less assaultive to my senses, but it was still there. Our ER was large but finite. It was hard to keep up with the patient load, but working in the department gave me moments, in the early mornings usually, when I could revel in the false security that I had it all under control. I knew who was in every room and what they were there for, and I had some inkling of whether they would need my help. My head was above water. By nine a.m., the illusion of orderliness was gone. The trickle of patients would become a torrent, or I would get sucked into a lengthy one-on-one intervention. The rest of the shift was a relentless scramble to keep up, to not miss something import-ant. But when the shift was over, it was over, and I got to start fresh the next day with new patients.

Patients get discharged, transferred, or admitted. If a patient you worked with was still in the ER when it was the end of your shift, you handed them off. There were no handoffs in my new role. The stack of paperwork, voicemails, and emails was always waiting for me, buried under new arrivals.

My first ER director would sometimes walk away from her desk to work a stint at triage. If we were well staffed with nurses, she might duck into rooms and offer coffee to visitors or cover patients with heated blankets. She said she did this for some instant gratification, when banging her head against the slow-moving wheels of administrative work was not meeting her need to make an immediate difference.

I remembered her saying this, because in that moment I swore to remember that I was lucky in this way; everything I did in those early days was in response to immediate needs and felt like it mattered to some extent on a personal level—the patient's and mine.

No matter how hard a day it was, I left feeling that I had made a difference. Even if it was a day of basic assistance, I had made an ER visit easier for patients and their families. Most days included tasks that were challenging and suited to my skills.

I couldn't resolve a housing situation, but I could find a shelter for that night and give resources for a longer-term solution. I couldn't change insurance coverage, but I could tell you where to get your antibiotic filled for free. I could not prevent your accident, but I could duck under the tubing in your arms and skirt around medical providers to hold a phone to your head so you could tell your mom you're OK. When your mom arrived, I'd get her to your bedside as quickly as possible.

I could not eliminate the disparities and inequities of our health care system, but I could put a Band-Aid on today's problem. Most days I went home feeling the reward of meeting nonstop challenges with some grace and kindness. But once I shifted gears to more administrative work, I lost that sense of closure and the satisfaction that the end of a shift brings.

I never guessed that I would be based in an office one day, grinding away alone, making calls to patients about mostly non-emergent matters, pushing applications through the hiring process, reviewing reports of child and elder abuse that someone else wrote, and listening to complaints about ER experiences.

The unanticipated stress of not working on the front lines came in the form of worth and value: Did my work still matter? This question was sparked by an internal drive—my own need for a sense of accomplishment and growth—but also an external concern. If you're not essential to the mission, you're fat. Fat gets trimmed out of hospital budgets all the time. I survived four ER directors and multiple budget cut cycles. I had to keep my job—I carried my family's health insurance.

Simple but Not Easy

Imagine, Act, Listen. Ideally the order would be: Listen, Imagine, Act. But who figures life out in an orderly way? My imagination was innate, acting was the job requirement, and listening—the bland tool that seemed the least powerful—got pushed to the side until I realized I was going in circles. If I wanted to go somewhere new, I needed to go deeper.

Becoming a good listener is Social Work 101: As you learn what it means to really listen, you realize that you've been failing at it your entire life. You strive to improve. You limit the damage of your measly skills by practicing on your fellow students. It requires work, a muscle to train and then flex over and over. The first test is whether you can hear, really hear, the feedback of those students, professors, and intern supervisors as they comment on your shortcomings.

It's about paying attention, giving your time, calming your ego, and releasing the desire for control. Even if you're determined to get better, you'll falter for quite a while. You start off awkwardly, nodding too much, inserting verbal encouragements too frequently, eager to build a connection with a client, hoping they will like you (but it is forbidden to wish that, so you never admit it).

For my bachelor's degree I interned at a private psychiatric hospital. My supervisor had me record an interaction with a new patient (with his permission). He was a middle-aged electrician having paranoid thoughts. His hair was long, his beard unkempt. He fidgeted in his chair. We were doing an intake interview so I could compile a social history report. Listening to the recording, my supervisor pointed out how often I responded, "You're right," to the patient's perspective of his situation. She asked me, "But is he really right?" I thought I was harmlessly signaling to him, "I understand. I get you." I hadn't intended to validate his belief system.

Once you graduate, maintenance of your listening skills is on you. If you're diligent, you prepare before you interact with a client, and later when alone, you reflect, though post-interaction reflection isn't always trustworthy. You may cast your performance in a warm softness, aglow with your brilliance, or you may smear it with muck, certain that it was the most inept work done by any social worker anywhere. I had both an inner critic and a sycophant to my ego, and they fought over what version to feed me.

I strove for more objectivity. I reflected on what was said and what was unsaid. I tried to imagine what I missed. I resolved to improve. My confidence in my listening skills grew. I assumed they would always be there for me.

$$\triangle$$

A client-centered approach means that the client defines the problem, and that's where the work starts. But the mission of the ER is to assess the patient for medical problems. Listening for nuances seemed a luxury we didn't have. Medical providers may start their assessment with what a patient says bothers them the most, but test results and findings (or lack thereof) can indicate a course of action independent of the patient's opinions.

If the patient didn't agree on the recommended course of action, there wasn't time to explore their thought processes, develop insight, and achieve a more organic and autonomous buy-in. We force-fed them the facts—our facts, sometimes to the neglect of their facts. We couldn't fully consider a systems view of the person in their environment, because we didn't have time for that. We rolled right over their "Yes, but."

In the scramble of Act, of always rushing to the next thing, doing whatever needed to be done, I'd failed to keep my listening skills strong. No one told me that those skills were in the "use it or lose it" category. Most of the listening I was doing was for peril: the charge nurse announcing a Level 2, the sound of an ambulance backing up in the bay, the wail of someone in terror.

My ears were attuned to the sound of red flags rustling and rationalizations humming in the air: from the patient who stayed with someone who hurt or neglected them, or from the family members omitting details of how a vulnerable patient had an inexplicable injury. Hearing what no one wanted to hear, that I could do. Though undoubtedly, I missed scores of such situations.

What was the effect of attuning my ears in this way? Did listening for lies, half-truths, and fear limit the spectrum of expression I could access? What does inviting suspicion into everyday listening do to your listening ability?

How I listened in the ER was a perversion of *why* I learned to listen as a social worker. I justified it by the ends—protection of the patient. It was a necessary focus, but when I needed to expand my listening skills, to hear more than risk and suspicion, my muscle was limp. I didn't know if the atrophy was due to my being stuck in danger-hunting mode or problem-solving mode, or if I'd grown complacent. I knew my bad listening habits had become worse. For instance, I interrupted, mentally rejecting the long answer as I felt the pressure of the next patient or staff member waiting on me, wanting to wrap up a conversation quickly to get to the next thing on my list.

Interruption comes naturally to me, being an impatient, talkative person. I listen with an agenda, plucking out the information I need, tuning out the extraneous. I was doing this at work—with patients, families, and staff—and I was doing this at home with my own family.

I valued my assessment, problem-solving, and resource-linking skills over my listening skills. It's part of why I was never interested in being a therapist, as much as I revere them. I don't want to sit and listen all day; I want to be doing. Each complaint I responded to was in danger of ending badly because I was gritting my way through it, willing myself to endure conversations that wound round and round with no exit in sight.

My motivation to change sprang from awareness of my own an-noyance. A nice person like me shouldn't be so annoyed so often with so little provocation. I wasn't annoyed at myself, of course. Oh, no! I was annoyed at *them*. So much unnecessary information. Why couldn't people just tell me what I needed to know? Why did we have to dance in circles when a straight line could get us there so much faster?

People like to tell stories. The social work profession raised me to hold space, make time, allow information to unravel at its own pace—to revere stories. But those ideals, and my personal love of stories, hit the brick wall of too many patients and not enough time, because something bigger and more urgent is always coming our way. Hurry up and finish this so you'll be ready for the next thing, which will probably take everything you've got.

Basically, I was asking everyone to be less human so I could clear my to-do list. *"Let's engage in a rote exchange of information so we can both just be on our way and not bother with a relationship."* I was far from that student who went into social work because she had a need to serve, to make a difference. People had become obstacles to surmount to complete a task, hash marks on the tally of the day's interventions. This is "emotional distancing," perceiving people as problems or ob-jects, part of the cynicism so often noted as an aspect of burnout.[1]

Common to both urgent and nonurgent patients is the complaint that we "didn't listen." The patient or family felt we were distracted, in too much of a hurry, or had made up our minds without regard for their perspective. Hearing them now, when they called back with their complaint, was essential.

A grievance is a problem with an experience in the past. There is no true resolution, no undoing what was done. The best you can usu-ally do is help the other person feel heard, be a witness to whatever bad thing happened (or they perceived happened) while in our ER. Being heard is a powerful gift that we rarely experience. It doesn't change

---

1. Jonathan Malesic, "How Men Burn Out," *New York Times*, January 4, 2022, https://www.nytimes.com/2022/01/04/opinion/burnout-men-signs.html.

what happened, but it can change how the patient or family member feels about the ER. If they believed I understood what they went through, our positive connection stood in contrast to their complaint.

In our work with families who'd experienced the trauma of a loved one critically injured or killed, our being tender with them, taking time to care for their needs, was a compassionate response that could have a lasting impact: imparting a memory to run alongside the traumatic one, how someone cared for them in that terrible time. It didn't change what happened, but it cushioned the wound.

A complaint isn't a trauma, but the person complaining is hurt, bewildered, or angry—something bad happened to them. Listening to such stories is what social workers do. It was now the main part of my job. I assumed my listening skills were still in place. I reached for them, tipping back into a trust fall, expecting to be caught in their waiting arms.

And I hit the floor hard.

$$\triangle$$

To reboot my listening skills, I settled on a self-study of the book *The Zen of Listening*, by Rebecca Z. Shafir. The book confirmed the reasons for my skills having grown rusty: complacency in my job, a frantic pace driving me toward impatience, and a preference to fix problems instead of "be" with them. And it added one I'd not considered—the complication of aging.

Being "only" in my fifties, I was resistant to this possibility. But even when there is no significant hearing impairment, listening gets harder as we age. There is a cognitive component to how we process conversations, especially if there are distractions—other speakers, background noise, comments that don't fit the context. Studies show that these are common obstacles for people as they get older.[2]

Lack of interest and concentration were other obstacles I had to

2. Sofie Degeest, Hannah Keppler, and Paul Corthals, "The Effect of Age on Listening Effort," *Journal of Speech, Language, and Hearing Research*, 58, no. 5 (2015): 1592–1600, https://doi.org/10.1044/2015_JSLHR-H-14-0288.

own. I had become a sloppy listener. I told myself that listening was no longer a ticket to get me to the main attraction; it *was* the main attraction. I didn't have to rush it. In fact, I mustn't rush it.

Now that all of my work was in an office, phone follow-ups had no competition from urgent issues. I didn't have to hurry through calls to get to a department full of patients. I had time to linger in conversations, even if I didn't want to. That was the job.

I could be good in a room. I could detect and address the nonverbal cues. As I reviewed resources for a patient's discharge plan, I might catch a head shake—an indication of some unknown obstacle—and say, "Looks like you don't think that's going to work." That head shake might be all you get, and on the phone it was invisible. To interpret silences and tone, I had to listen more closely.

Without the nonverbal cues I'd pick up from being in a room with someone, how could I know if the patient was receptive to our urging to see a specialist? If they understood the possible consequences of not testing their blood sugar or seeing a dietician for diabetes, or of not going to physical therapy for an ankle injury? Were they following my explanation of why we didn't do the test they wanted, or were they flinging an "eat shit" look at me that I couldn't catch over the phone?

In *The Zen of Listening*, there's a test for assessing your listening abilities. Out of a possible score of 25, I got a 17.5. This put me in the category of a "good listener." Reporter bias was likely.

The test identified particular behaviors that could be barriers to better listening, including a tendency to observe and judge at the same time, focusing on outcome, and being distracted by a hidden agenda. Guilty on all counts. Adverse conditions, including hostile customers or coworkers, add to listening difficulties because the need to build up our defenses distracts us from processing the message. Anxiety also impacts our ability to listen mindfully. Check, check, and check.

There are no easy cures, though Shafir outlines helpful methods to enhance your focus on the person talking. Regarding concentration, she maintains that we need "intent and interest." She urges readers to cultivate a curiosity about the person and a willingness to believe that any verbal encounter can contain something valuable.

Grievance management requires stillness, shifting out of problem-solving mode, armed with only one Band-Aid—the listening itself. The only reward (besides keeping my job) was the sliver of hope that I could end a conversation on a good note, with a positive connection. This served the hospital, but it also served me and the patient.

"Silence is sharing," says Shafir.[3] I found that the more I slowed down the pace of conversation, the more often silences occurred. Often the hardest things are said after a period of silence, in the gaps that we leave between the routine phrases we lean on. Respecting those gaps signals patience, a willingness to stay and listen even when the content grows sparse and uneven. *"Is there anything else? I have the time."*

I didn't need a script. My attentive silence said it all.

△

Mrs. Roberts came in for elevated blood pressure and was discharged to follow up with her primary care physician to be assessed for a possible medication change. She felt that the visit was a waste of time and money and that the nurse discounted her concerns.

I spoke with her over the phone: "I'm so sorry. Can you help me understand what the nurse did or said that made you feel that way?"

"She acted like my blood pressure was no big deal and even said, 'That's not that bad. I've seen much higher.'"

"So, did it seem to you that she didn't take your concern seriously?"

"Yes, because why on earth would I be there if there wasn't a problem?"

"Sure. You took your pressure at home, and it was really high."

"Yes."

"And it was still high when you got to the ER."

"That's right, and she saw it!"

"You know, as a social worker I don't have medical training, but I've learned that blood pressure rates vary widely; what is high for you may be normal for someone else, and your blood pressure rate that day

---

3. Rebecca Shafir, *The Zen of Listening* (Quest Books, 2000).

may have been your highest, but the nurse has seen many that were much higher. But I understand it was high for you—that's why you came in. I think she knew that, and I'm sorry she didn't say it. Maybe she was trying to reassure you, knowing that you were worried."

"No, she wasn't trying to make me feel better; she just didn't think I should be there."

"OK. Well, I do see that she hooked you up to a monitor to keep an eye on your blood pressure and called your pharmacy to make sure we had the right information about your medication. And that our doctor called your doctor to let her know you were here, and to make sure that you could follow up the next day. We gave you an EKG to check your heart and gave you fluids. But I'll let the nurse know how you feel. I know that she would not want you to think that she didn't take you seriously . . . Is there anything else you want to tell me?"

(Silence as I wait for it.) There was something else. Another strike against the nurse was that she asked the required screening question for domestic abuse. "She asked me if I felt safe at home!"

"Yes, we have to ask everyone that now, men and women, even children if they're old enough to answer us."

"Well, I've never been asked that before."

"We've been doing that for two years, and it's not just us; every hospital is supposed to ask that question."

"Are they gonna ask me again, if I come back?"

"Yes, they're supposed to ask every time because your situation could always change, and if you are in danger we want to know so we can help."

Mrs. Roberts ended our conversation on a pleasant note, saying she appreciated my call, and I said I appreciated the feedback and would share it with the nurse. She sounded satisfied and told me to have a good evening.

Patients and families often had perceptions about staff that I felt were misunderstandings. I could vouch for a doctor or staff member, but not until I listened and imagined, until I could view the experience through the patient's eyes, understand the issue, and sincerely commiserate.

Explanations are not usually helpful. Regardless of even gentle reasoning, a patient would still feel that we should have done that MRI, minimized their waiting time, or given them a referral that worked better for their unique situation. The person complaining was so immersed in the stew of emotions evoked by our conversation that anything I might provide by way of an explanation sounded like an excuse.

The truth is I often thought we could do better, but I felt compelled to offer the patient or family a glimpse into the ER side of their experience on the chance that it might help them understand our process, how we make decisions. I hoped to educate them as well as depersonalize whatever had occurred. But this could only happen if I first gained insight into their perspective and believably communicated my understanding.

I couldn't always gauge their openness to our perspective, so I just said, "I have some information that might shed some light on this, but I don't know if that would be helpful to you right now." Usually they told me to proceed, and then found reasons why, in their case, we should have made an exception.

Sometimes the information I gave seemed to make a difference during our conversation. It didn't cure them of their anger or their insistence that we should have done something differently, but they saw the picture from our perspective, making their memory of the experience less personally offensive.

Using my skills to develop a rapport with patients for the public relations benefit of a corporation felt like selling out on my social work values. But I decided that as long as I put the patient first, I was on solid ground.

Once, my adult son came over for dinner and asked me about my day. I gave him the general outline of three complaints I'd worked on: A wife thought her husband waited too long to be seen, especially since he ended up being admitted; a patient thought the doctor should have ordered a CT scan for his chronic back pain; and a man objected to the tone of voice security staff used when he tried to get back to his sister's room (the patient already had three visitors, but none were willing to step out). I must have channeled the patients' point of view, because he asked, "So, you take the patients' side?"

I wasn't sure what to say. For me to take sides meant I believed that someone was right and someone was wrong. It was rarely that simple. I didn't see it as "taking sides," but many ER staff members reacted to my patient advocacy as a betrayal of our team. They felt that I chose to believe a patient over them, whereas I felt my mission was comparable to theirs—to serve the patient by putting them first. Through grievances we can learn ways to improve service and care and increase safety; I felt my work helped to protect all our jobs by making the hospital better.

Medical staff feared criticism about their technical skill, but medical skills were almost never the focus of a complaint. Doctors and staff were accused of being dismissive, rude, rushed, and biased. I'm sure they were sometimes, but I also know that to be a patient is to feel vulnerable, that vulnerability is uncomfortable, and that discomfort activates vigilance and sensitivity.

A feeling of vulnerability exists in ER patients regardless of how sick they are. Coming to the ER is an admission of need—whatever is going on with you has exceeded your ability to deal with it. Crossing our threshold is a request for help, and asking for help is humbling. And into this humble moment we rush in.

We subject you to a sorting system that you don't understand and can't influence. We undress you; we do things that hurt and expose you to risk—all with no guarantee that you are going to leave feeling better.

Even if we succeed in making you better or finding a diagnosis, if we fail to reassure you or earn your confidence, you're more likely to complain. Once you're feeling stronger and safer, you're ready to strike back.

△

Sometimes a complaint came from a patient who had been admitted. If I received the complaint before they left the hospital, I tried to meet the patient and family in person. This came with inherent tension—I might walk right into a frenzy of accusations, trapped in a small room, pelted with questions I couldn't fully anticipate.

The nurses and staff up on the floor unit often stood in the doorway when I made my visit, curious to see how I would handle the issue the patient or family had been reliving since arriving from the ER. Far from my home department, I didn't assume this staff had my back. They were not my team and likely had their own complaints with the ER: the way we transferred patients to them right when they wanted to go to lunch, the way we had treated their family when they came to the ER as patients, their annoyance at the ER swagger—self-important, confident, and thriving amid chaos.

ER staff believes they are the redheaded stepchild of the hospital—misunderstood and unsupported. I didn't want to have a chip on my shoulder, but I perceived the floor staff as licking their lips, eager to watch me get ripped apart.

Despite my fear, I learned that no amount of information gathering or strategizing ahead of time was helpful to surviving such encounters. It didn't matter how much I knew. The weapons of argument were left at the door. The goal was not to convince the patient or family of anything except my willingness to listen. Humiliation was a strong possibility, but humility was the key. I took accusations on the chin yet threw no blows. I listened. I said, "I'm sorry." I felt vulnerable. But it wasn't the same as their vulnerability—I wasn't hurt or sick, and neither was my family.

Those meetings usually went well. I doubt I changed anyone's mind about their experience or influenced their ratings on the patient survey, but these interactions served as my quick fix. In the same way my director craved the instant gratification of leaving her desk to bring a patient a warm blanket, I liked leaving my desk to show up for a patient and family. They appreciated the effort. The inpatient staff found it gratifying that the department at fault came to take responsibility. As

Eckhart Tolle writes, "Being present is always infinitely more powerful than anything one could say or do."[4]

△

I continued with case management follow-ups at this time, and they held their own challenge. Case management calls resembled the structure of making rounds to ER rooms: me in the role of problem seeker, directing a strategic conversation about the obstacles keeping the patient from the resources they needed. It could be more fulfilling than complaint management, but also more discouraging.

Complaint management had a redeeming feature: It was an intervention with three acts—listen, explore, apologize. Most complaints ended after that third act, and our goodbyes were usually friendly, with the comradery of a shared experience. There was a sense of satisfied completion, a file I could shut. I never had to revisit that particular complaint and was unlikely to speak with that patient again—we were both moving on.

But case management was a never-ending serial soap opera, minus the romance. You could go a year without tuning in, come back, and pick up right where you left off—tons of patients made multiple visits. Nothing visibly changed.

I tried to find encouragement in the reduced visits of some patients I followed up with. But I wasn't built to correlate success with the absence of an event—a lower number of visits seemed as likely to be due to random chance as to my intervention. Still, the data was there. It could allay fears of losing my job, but it didn't infuse my work with meaning.

The list of names of patients making numerous visits was overwhelming, and often included those who wanted something I couldn't give them—treatment for their pain. Patients who made the frequent-visit list included those with a history of coming in with pain

---

4. Eckhart Tolle, *A New Earth* (Plume Books, 2006), 176.

complaints and requests for specific pain medications. I contacted them to hear their story and offer resources, sometimes referring them to pain clinics. I explained why the ER could not prescribe such medications. I didn't agonize over who was drug-seeking and whose pain was "legit." Pain is pain. My work was the same regardless of the story: listen, empathize, and refer.

These were hard stories to hear: the construction worker who hurt his back from a fall and couldn't work, the young mother whose neck pain never left after a car accident. Sometimes the source of the pain wasn't known, despite X-rays and tests. If there was a possible cure—surgery, physical therapy, or medication—these patients couldn't afford it. Rarely did anyone admit addiction. But family members sometimes outed patients.

We'd get calls when the patients were being treated or following a visit. Families begged us to make a note in their loved one's chart about what they believed was addiction, hoping we'd agree to never again prescribe them a pain medication. Families might launch into a complaint about how doctors got the patient into this predicament to begin with by issuing generous prescriptions in response to an injury or illness.

We couldn't comment to the family member about the patient's care. We offered them what we offered the patients—referrals, support, and the harsh outline of our process: A new assessment is made each visit. The doctor's disposition may or may not include medication, depending on the assessment. We could make no promises. A patient's problem could change, and our actions shift in response to what the doctor finds. But if we knew a patient had a history of requesting pain medication, they would be unlikely to receive a prescription for a controlled substance.

When making follow-up calls to patients, my biggest listening challenge was to quiet my bias. There can be a place for calling out bullshit, but it requires a certainty about a patient that we rarely have in the ER. I could listen freely, because unlike medical providers, my beliefs would not impact a treatment decision. I didn't have to worry about being manipulated; I didn't have the power to write a prescription.

My job required me to frequently ask physicians for help: to make a referral to specialists, to run tests they hadn't planned on, to reconsider a patient for admission, to return to a treatment room to answer questions or respond to new concerns. But when it came to pain medication, the most I would do is relay the patient's story and communicate their request to the doctor. I usually left my opinion, my advocacy, out of it. I didn't, and couldn't, know the truth of how they were using pain medication, and the consequences of being wrong were too risky.

Too much medicine can feed an addiction, fuel drug selling, or play a part in an overdose. It can reinforce the tendency to come to the ER, which drains our resources, doesn't help the patient in the long run, and hurts other patients needing our assistance. And there are risks to the doctor as well: Prescribing pain medication brings a doctor under scrutiny. Yet too little medicine results in suffering.

All I had to offer was compassion and information. And they were welcome to that regardless of where they were located on the addiction continuum—if they were on it at all. On my follow-up calls, I listened for the parts in their story where I might help. I didn't doubt their difficulty in finding a provider to help them; many came to the ER as a last resort. Sometimes it was a last resort due to a consequence of their behavior and choices—exhausting their providers by frequent visits and requests.

Patients have told me they were "fired" by their doctor. I've seen the official letters stating they were no longer welcome in a doctor's practice, that the doctor assumes no further obligation toward them. I didn't waste time choosing sides, defending the patient or the doctor, because it was beside the point—we were obligated to see the patient each time they came in. They could always come here, but they may not get what they were looking for.

In the early aughts, prescription drug monitoring programs became established in most states, including Georgia. This allowed physicians to look up a patient and see their prescription history of controlled substances. They could detect potential "ER shopping" with objective data, rather than relying on a patient's honesty or memory. As opioid abuse spread, it became more common to hear doctors explain to the patients they were discharging why over-the-counter medications were preferable to a prescription.

At that point, the ER was seeing over two hundred patients a day. I continued to make my calls to patients who made the frequent-visit list. Those patients may have seen a different doctor each visit. The ER doesn't have the continuity and familiarity that a regular provider has with their patients; we can't prescribe narcotic painkillers partly because we can't monitor the use.

It's easy to agree with these patients that the health care system is a mess, that too many people fall into the wide gaps of care. Whether their need stems from addiction, chronic pain, or a combination of both, there is too much suffering with too little help.

To some patients, my empathy rang hollow, if they even perceived me as empathetic. I was another person "firing" them from care. I assured them that they could always come to the ER, we would always see and evaluate them, but also remarked that it was unlikely their request for pain medication would be met.

Often the frequency of their visits lessened after my follow-up call, at least for a while. Maybe they found a provider, maybe they went to another ER, or maybe they were just suffering quietly, holding off until they couldn't take it anymore.

When the visits increased again and they went back on my list, they wouldn't answer my calls, or if they did, they were defensive, bristling at my interference. I would ask if they had tried the resources I had given them, wanting to identify and resolve obstacles to getting them care. This was "Yes, but" territory: "Yes," they knew the options, "but" they had endless reasons why those options wouldn't work for them.

Usually I wouldn't call them again unless they had a new problem, because I'd become the ER police—in their eyes and in my own—instead of someone trying to help. I'd become their new obstacle. I didn't dare risk discouraging them from a future visit. The ER might be their best option for whatever care they might need in the future.

"The patient comes first" is a maxim you hear throughout the hospital. When the best thing for the ER matched the best thing for the patient, my work was easy. But often they didn't match. What was at stake for the individual patient had to be more important to me than what was at stake for the hospital. I reminded myself that I was a helper, not a gatekeeper.

Last Shifts

Although I've always been someone who writes, I didn't journal much about the ER. I was plagued by images and feelings from the work, so I assumed I would remember it all whether I wanted to or not. When I started in the ER at twenty-eight, I didn't really know how memory worked (or didn't work), how events shape-shift, how wrestling hard things into the deep doesn't keep them down but causes them to float up, blurry and sticky.

I came to understand that having a clearer hold on my memories made them easier to process. The monster I *imagined* under the bed was much more disturbing than what I found when I looked directly at it. When my work shifted away from direct patient care, I recognized it was an ending of sorts, a transition, and I wanted to make sense of it. Did those years working at the bedside of patients mean anything to me beyond a trial by fire, a crash course on surviving trauma and mayhem?

My usual journaling focused on the creative aspect of my life: noting the impact of art, nature, films, books, dreams; sorting out relationship dynamics to glean insight that would, I hoped, drive personal growth. But as the shift work began winding down, it seemed that I was going to survive it after all, and actually miss it. I wanted to remember what I could. It was a tunnel, not a cave, and I could see the light at the end of it. I loosened my compartmentalizing barriers and invited the ER to come into my off time.

Through journaling, I try to purge myself of the callous, cavalier tone that rattles on in my head. I feel passionate, anguished, energized, and rewarded by the work, but every job, no matter how perverse, becomes normalized with time. You develop routine desires: You want a shift where you get to take your lunch break, one where your feet won't hurt six hours in with six more hours to go; you want to be there when someone brings in a cake, or donuts, or anything unexpected, free, and full of sugar; and you want a shift where nobody dies.

Here are some excerpts from my journal on some last shifts.

In this first one, I felt guilty about wanting an easy shift for the wrong reason. At times I felt like the caustic nurse on some medical show who orders a patient not to die because "it's too much paperwork."

> *Having an easy shift means it's not too busy, not too slow, no one is too awful to me, there's no thorny problems that ravage me emotionally, and no one dies. I want this for myself. What about the people actually impacted? If things go badly, I have a rough shift, but their life is upended.*

I was also aware of my detachment:

> *Ten-year-old comes out of a room sobbing, and the nurse manager standing beside me bursts into tears. The boy is the son of a patient, his father was a pedestrian hit by a car. The dad is probably going to die when he gets up to ICU. This may be the son's last time seeing him.*
>
> *The nurse's reaction caught me by surprise. Yes, it's desperately sad, but her tears are foreign, a language I no longer recognize. I only look at her for a moment before I realize that I am the odd one: When was the last time I burst into tears spontaneously? And will I ever do that again?*
>
> *I've been beside this family throughout this traumatic event. I wasn't sure that bringing the child into the room was the right decision, but that was what they*

wanted, and I respected their judgment. I talked to him before he went in and rushed to comfort him when he came out alone, as the rest of his family stayed in the room.

It was extremely sad, but I did it all without shedding a single tear, whereas Alice had waterworks as soon as she saw the son. Appalled at my restraint, I did a little body check, maybe there was something . . . just under the surface, under one layer, two layers? Checking, checking . . . I find only dry-eyed compassion.

It's selfish to make this about me, but that's the point of writing it. Everything about claiming space for yourself, observing, and lamenting the impact on you feels selfish in the face of the actual tragedy others are living. I worry that I am just going through the motions, so well tuned is my ability to emotionally detach. Occupational hazard.

I reflected on the ongoing emotional burden of deaths:

I bury them deep, but they linger on in my brain tissue, in the chronic clenching of my jaw, leading to one tooth extraction with a risk of four more.

I have become hypervigilant when I'm near the front doors—watching for the next person to bust through the door, a small limp body draped over his arms. Because that has happened and will again.

And then there are the dreams, so that even if I'm far away from the ER, and days from my last shift, the experience still finds me.

During this time when my shift work was winding down, I worked three deaths in which the only family member to come to the ER was the surviving spouse. All three patients were elderly women. I worked other deaths that year, other cases that were more sensational, but these three happened within a couple of months of each other, and each struck a deeper chord of sadness than I usually felt in the expected deaths of the elderly.

In my fifties then, perhaps this reaction was part of my developmental shift. For so many years my fears were for my children, or even for my own life, as I worried about the impact of my potential death before they were grown. Now, in these losses of longtime partners, I saw what the future held for me or my husband.

Older men, newly made widowers, are the worst for coming to the ER alone, following the ambulance that carries their bride of so many years. They don't tell any family or friends that they've come, and they won't let me call anyone for them. I stay close. We sit together quietly, the doctor comes in, speaks briefly, the doctor goes out. I get them to their wife's side, and then I walk them out. They get into their cars alone to go back to that empty house stained with the evidence of the event that changed their life.

One time the neighbors came. He did not call them; he told me there was no one to call, which is what all these old men say. The neighbors saw the ambulance. They knew he came alone and would be here all alone.

I love these neighbors. I love what their coming says about them, about humanity in general, but if I'm honest, I also love them for me. They soften the hardness of my memory. I don't know how much the neighbors really help the widower, but they damn sure help me.

△

Psychologist Erik Erikson's stage of development for age forty to sixty-five is Generativity vs. Stagnation.[1] He says that if we complete this stage successfully, we learn the value of *care.* This is caring that extends to your community or to the next generation; it's bigger than parenting or caring for your parents. This is his next to last stage.

A good manager cares and therefore must be curious about the personal lives of those she supervises, about their families, their struggles, about how the work contributes to their goals and needs or subtracts from them. Unlike the patients that you gear up for, interact with, and leave, you work with these people daily or weekly. The quality of your interactions depends on a positive foundation—you can't fake it.

In my fifteen years managing the group of advocates, I tried to get their salaries increased, provide them professional growth opportunities, and have their role become a more respected part of the ER team. I succeeded here and there, but as time went on, the successes became fewer and fewer. I was banging my head against an institution that didn't recognize their value or at least wasn't willing to fully compensate it. As the hospital became part of a corporate, bigger medical system, roles became more delineated, each fitting into a rigid category. Advocates were a unique ER role in an organization that now wanted people with cookie-cutter skills they understood and could plug into standardized positions. Support for a yearly retreat, an educational workshop, and even regular meetings was withdrawn.

A unique role calls for workers that don't always fit the mold. Advocates were hired for their blend of compassion and practicality, for having good judgment and knowing how to direct it autonomously, for having people skills to use with patients and staff, and for not being easily spooked.

With benefits, job security, and a guarantee of interesting work, being an ER advocate can be a good place to land, especially if you don't stay too long. It takes a particular sort of person to do the job. We found experienced social workers looking to supplement their salaries, undergraduates looking for relevant experience, stay-at-home moms

---

1. Erik Erikson, *Childhood and Society* (W. W. Norton & Company, 1950), 268.

returning to the workforce, and people of all ages wanting to make a difference. Many incredible people did time in the ER as advocates before going on with their lives in new directions, and it was an honor to know them.

The advocates were almost always women; the occasional man was usually either a graduate student or supplementing his income. Two hires, one male and one female, were pre-med and later became doctors. I know working as a patient advocate gave them each an incomparable experience to bring to their practice, to their patients, and to their worldview.

The easiest hires, in terms of choosing them, training them, and managing them, were social workers who had worked for the state. They often came from the Division of Family and Children Services, frequently in child protection. Working a stint with the state meant that they knew how to work hard, regardless of the difficulty and low pay, were familiar with the community's resources, and understood that their successes and failures could directly impact lives. They did not scare easily.

Some just worked relief or part-time for us; others left their state jobs completely to work with us full-time. They told me how good it felt to be appreciated, to have people say thank you even for something small. I still wanted improvements, but it reminded me that there were harder jobs and darker places.

Even the advocates who felt positive about the work struggled against the conditions. Hired into a schedule of assigned shifts, they were stuck with that schedule until someone quit, working hours and days that might no longer be compatible with their lives. Shifts were physically demanding despite how you felt that day—if being on your feet hurt, you were going to be in pain for hours. There were now fewer opportunities for professional growth, and advocates were always underpaid.

Similar to how I couldn't effect change with our most frequent patients, I couldn't sustain the effort of trying to make things better for the advocates. I was up against a system entrenched in survival mode, pushing for delivery of services for the least amount of cost, even at the risk of losing employees. ER directors were supportive of the advocate role, at least in theory, seeing value in the services we provided for patients and in the easing of the nurses' load of nonmedical tasks. We also had the support of the doctors, who pulled us back from the brink of budget cuts many times.

ER doctors are resource savvy. With too much to do for too many patients, and with nurses and techs overwhelmed with medical tasks, they looked to us to gather information from patients, families, nursing homes, and community resources. They trusted us to interpret history given by family members, to make assessments of child and elder abuse and domestic violence, to obtain needed resources, and to join them in rooms where something hard had to be said.

But despite the support of the doctors and directors, the needs of advocates weren't met in the fundamental ways needed to ensure the long-term health of the role and the individuals.

In the early years of management, I had this quote on my office wall:

> Barbara Meier: What are the rewards?
>
> Jerry Garcia: Mainly the rewards of service. It's a simple thing, the feeling of a job well done. There's a workmanlike quality that depends, I'm sure, on the same sensibility that makes the tea ceremony work, that kind of ritual of doing some simple task over and over again. It's not a big thing, but it's strong and important.[2]

I wanted the big and important work we had to do to be enough, for the rewards of service to compensate for our low pay. But this quote felt outdated and insensitive as I failed to get good people working an impossible job the support they needed to sustain themselves. A good manager cares, but caring too much without the power to change things made me miserable.

---

2. Barbara Meier, "Jerry Garcia Speaks with Barbara Meier," *Tricycle: The Buddhist Review*, Spring 1992, https://tricycle.org/magazine/jerry-garcia-speaks-with -barbara-meier/.

Part of a new administration's attempt to improve morale was a hospital-wide satisfaction survey for all employees. I was rated by my employees, and I received some negative comments indicating that I was an obstacle to improving their conditions and insensitive to their needs. Even though it was just a few comments from a couple of people, managers were told they must openly accept such remarks as deficits without excuse or objection and create an improvement plan that those workers found agreeable.

To stay in my job meant having to pretend that I was willing to work harder, that I didn't resent the hundreds of hours accrued for paid time off that I could never take, the holidays not spent with my family, and the toll of the ER on my well-being. I would have to pretend that I could do better, which meant I would have to lie. As I saw it, the hospital not only wanted me to lie, but to betray myself. I handed my boss my letter of resignation.

None of the issues listed by those advocates were things I could own. The real problem was both bigger and more basic: I no longer cared enough. How could I rehabilitate myself out of that? In making work only about work, I'd compartmentalized myself right out of my emotions. I did care about the advocates I supervised, even the disgruntled ones, but I didn't have the energy to engage, to teach, to defend the efforts I'd made and try again to change our circumstances. I was defeated in every way.

According to Deb Dana, author of *Anchored*, when you are stuck in a place of "going through the motions, drained of energy, disconnected, losing hope, giving up," you are functioning in the shutdown part of your autonomic nervous system.[3] I felt like a turtle retreating deep into my shell.

My boss was upset by my resignation; she felt that she had failed me. Her tears helped me forgive myself. She realized that she had resisted much of what I pushed for, what I knew the advocate group needed, yet I was paying the price and taking the blame. I had asked for more relief staff to facilitate requests for time off, for regular meetings

---

3. Deb Dana, *Anchored: How to Befriend Your Nervous System Using Polyvagal Theory* (Sounds True, 2021), 6.

and the occasional workshop, and, persistently, an increase in pay. But these requests would have impacted the department's budget. They were frills.

I could no longer be a part of the advocate team I had created. I wouldn't ever work another shift, and I wouldn't supervise the advocates. Surely I had to leave, because what else could I do? My boss offered me a way to stay. She valued my work in follow-ups and grievance management and wanted it to continue. I had mixed feelings about the proposition, knowing I would miss patient care and that I wouldn't be able to shake off the negativity of this transition. My connection to the advocates was irrevocably broken—how strange it would be to be one floor away from them but never again be a direct part of their lives and their work.

I could have left to try something else. But the ER was the devil I knew, and I still preferred that devil to the unknown. As a fifty-five-year-old, I wasn't up to the challenge of selling myself to get hired, learning a new job, and adjusting to new people. I also knew that the pay rate I'd aged into, my insurance and benefits, was unlikely to be matched, even now with my working fewer hours. Money and security were still a major factor, just like twenty-seven years before, when I first took the job.

My job got smaller. I reeled my curiosity in further. Since I'd now have even less power, it was better not to know what was and was not happening with individuals and with the role I had shaped and nurtured. Relentless caring was no longer a requirement I couldn't reach. I could choose whom to care about and I kept the list short, reversing any gains I'd made in Erikson's Generativity stage.

No longer working on the front lines meant that I'd kept the vow I made to myself when I got the job at the ER—I never fell out. Most of the medical staff never knew the extent of my issue, how nervous I was those first years, until I learned my triggers and concocted ways to work around them. That small success gave me no satisfaction.

Doing a "good job" was more than surviving and hiding my weaknesses. It meant making a difference, but to whom? The further I got from direct patient care, the more intangible that difference was. I worked in support of a department within a system. I believed in the mission of that department and in the system, but I was just a tiny part of a vast structure thundering down worn tracks that went in a circle.

When I started, I had a sort of reverence for the hospital. I believed its noble mission to help people in need must mean that those running it were so committed to that mission that they put it before their desires or obligations to make money. Yes, I was that naive.

A few years in, I got a peek behind the curtain. Some of the men throwing the big switches were so flawed that they knocked the hospital right off the pedestal I'd constructed. It felt personal; they betrayed my faith in them, in the mission.

I understand the temptation to condemn—the human response to cast an object of our disillusionment into a pit of opposite characteristics: If it isn't the best, it must be the worst. But I suspected this tendency within myself was another trick of perception. When the hospital failed to live up to my ideals, I decided my ideals were unrealistic.

I adjusted my expectations early on in my career: A place is only as good as its people. Good people come and go, along with the not so good. A hospital is an ever-changing entity, trying in vain to escape the fate it's condemned to by our country. I was now serving that entity more directly, shoveling coals into a ravenous mouth that wouldn't even miss me when I was gone. Someone would pick up my shovel, and the system would continue to chug along.

"Remember: Just because you're necessary doesn't mean you're important." This is on a poster with a cogwheel, produced by Despair, Inc., a company that parodies the banal slogans of corporate America. But my favorite poster of theirs shows a Mesoamerican temple pyramid with steep steps climbing to a sacrificial platform. It reads: "All we ask here is that you give us your heart."

△

In my journal, I included the time that Paula came in and got admitted. We were both fifty-five years old.

My mother-in-law had died, and so had my father. Our children were in college and living on their own. I was making time to write. My body determined tennis to be too damaging, but I found mountain biking. Life wasn't as busy; we made frequent trips to see my mother but also got away to camp close to biking trails.

Paula's life had changed too—she was getting worse. She still came in frequently, but now, as soon as she was conscious, she lunged off the bed to leave and often fell. Falls are problematic for a hospital. We are, of course, concerned about the patient getting injured on our watch— we take our responsibility to keep patients safe very seriously. But once falls began to generate automatic penalties, hospitals worked harder to find solutions.

Falls became one of the safety measures that hospitals are judged on—for ratings, for accreditation, for meeting standards that allow them to receive government monies. This motivates hospitals to document outcomes and incidents and come up with proactive measures. When a patient who falls frequently is also a patient who comes frequently, it trashes your safety score. Thus a "Paula protocol" was born.

First, we tried increasing our usual efforts: She'd go to a room close to the nurses' station. As she got fluids and sobered up, her nurse, techs, the advocate, and sometimes security staff all kept an eye and an ear out. Her door was left open. She continued to get up out of bed and fall.

We tried something new. We took the mattress off the gurney and put it on the floor. We cleared the room of the rolling stools and bedside stands. Falling was made almost impossible, because to fall, she would have to get up. Usually, she did not have enough coordination to do it, at least in the early part of the visit. We still kept her close and under a watchful eye. It worked, but no one liked it; it felt disrespectful.

Despite her many years of coming to the ER regularly, Paula still evoked more compassion than anger. Among the staff I started with, only a few were still working in the ER, but it didn't take long for new staff to get to know Paula. For nurses and techs, the frustration of caring for her was undeniable—no matter how busy you were you had to devote a large amount of attention to her to prevent her from getting injured. The damage of her lifestyle on her body and the futility of any hope for positive change could lead you to despair, if you let yourself dwell on it.

I didn't let myself dwell on it. I'd given up on her and on the many patients whose frequent visits continued for years despite my intervening multiple times to help them find services, such as follow-up care, shelter, or mental health services. A force of one, I had toiled away on these cases mostly without success. I knew something of their issues and their lives, and when staff complained about them being here yet again ("Can't case management do something?"), I reviewed their chart and updated their file to reflect resources we should continue to offer them. I shared this information with the staff, but unless there was a new resource needed or available, I no longer made dozens of phone call attempts, sent letters, tried to meet them on their visits, or went home with them—as I had done with Paula over ten years ago.

I'd seen Paula many times after that visit to her home, and when I didn't see her, I read about her in shift reports. I scanned her chart for indications that she needed or wanted something that I could provide.

Frequent ER users, just like everyone else, only got admitted if they were too unstable for discharge or if staying in the hospital meant they'd get an essential treatment that they couldn't receive outside of the hospital. Being unable to afford the essential treatment didn't usually satisfy the criteria. Paula was no longer rebounding the way she used to. She was still eager to leave as soon as possible, but finally she was too sick to insist.

ER staff is so accustomed to seeing these patients that come frequently that we forget they are unknown outside of our department. The inpatient staff caring for them and the physicians assigned to them are shocked when they look at the medical record and see the long list of ER visits over the years.

I'd never known Paula to be admitted before, so I alerted the inpatient social work department. I told them her basic issues and her long history. Perhaps her health had worsened to the point where she was incompetent to make her own care decisions, a finding that could result in her receiving care despite her objections.

By virtue of admission to the hospital, she was forced into sustained sobriety. They tried to place her for drug and alcohol treatment, but she refused, demanding to go home. The psychiatric RN evaluated her and found her competent to make her own decisions. She was discharged. Nothing changed. We didn't see her for a few weeks.

Then she was found dead in her home.

All we had in common was our age and gender and that our families loved us. Paula's family would still pick her up from the ER, and they came to see her during her stay on the floor. Paula and I only crossed paths because we both did time in the world of worst-case scenarios. But I got paid to be there. She was living in that realm 24/7. I had tried to get her out and I had failed.

Not long before Paula died, a nurse told me of seeing her for an unusual ER visit. She didn't arrive unconscious by ambulance; she walked in by choice for a minor problem. She wasn't drunk or in a blood sugar–related crisis. More of a customer than a patient for that visit, she sat upright on the mattress, and the mattress stayed on the gurney. She was fully dressed and made-up, and said thank you!

We marveled that a different Paula existed outside of our perception, forgetting that we only see a small slice of a person when they are a patient—even if we see them weekly for decades.

No one speculated that she'd stopped drinking or started taking her medication as recommended. Hope is a reckless choice in the ER. She was just having a relatively good day. We had forgotten that we only knew her on her worst days.

I regretted that I missed the chance to meet this other Paula. I'd so thoroughly given up on her making a change that it didn't even occur to me that what I should have regretted was missing a real opportunity to talk to her about her health. To try again. To risk a reckless hope.

A Need to Know

I have never been a particularly curious person. This seems at odds with having a vibrant imagination, but I think it's my brain's way of keeping stimulation at a manageable level—I'm already producing enough content on my own.

The hospital teaches employees not to snoop, or it tries to. Now that the chart is electronic, it can be audited, checked to see which staff looked at whose records. Confidentiality is a big deal; violations will get you fired.

I utilized a need-to-know criterion for anything happening on my shift. Just because you're there when a patient comes in doesn't mean you need to know all about them. If my shift partner had an interesting case on their section of the ER, I only needed to know what they needed to tell me. I read my coworkers' shift reports, and offered supportive comments on the hard cases, but I didn't ask many questions.

This wasn't just to comply with policy; it was self-protection. There were already too many things I had to know that I didn't want to know. Every shift served me a lifetime's worth of trauma and horror. Why seek more? I sought only to know what I must know, putting me at odds with some of my coworkers, who seemed to have an endless capacity for the drama of trauma.

△

In a pod of offices one flight up from the ER, coworkers in the office next to me talked about an accident. In our line of work, accidents are expected. I only perked up because a bicycle was mentioned, and my husband and I bike.

In the lingo used by medics, this accident was "bike vs. car." That is not a fair fight. This sort of tagline—train vs. car, car vs. eighteen-wheeler, car vs. pedestrian—drops you right into the arena of the accident scene. In your mind's eye you size up the two sides as if they are prize fighters. But where a smaller fighter may benefit from speed and agility, in crashes, pure brawn wins the day. You have to imagine the winner. The loser lies before you on the gurney.

This EMS report stated: *The bike was in pieces, lights still flashing though it was daylight,* perhaps making the point that the cyclist had had her lights on as an extra safety precaution. *Her clothes were torn and bloody.*

Two of my husband's cycling friends have died while biking. The cyclist in this report on my coworker's desk was still alive. She had gone to surgery and sounded stable. The only question I asked was where it happened.

She was hit on a congested main road where I bike, headed to a park that I go to. She was only a year younger than me. I drew these connections aloud. My coworkers listened in.

"What was a woman her age doing riding a bike on that street with all that traffic?" I said with mock indignation. My coworkers narrowed their eyes, not sure if I knew that I was describing myself. I laughed. They joined in a little nervously.

They realized I was making fun of myself but were a bit uncomfortable because certainly they'd had such thoughts about me; possibly they'd had this exact conversation when I wasn't in the office. One of them said to me, "Yeah, it's like she took the hit for you."

That was a sickening thought. I didn't look up this patient's chart; I had no legit "need to know." I was just curious. But in the absence of facts, I imagined that she recovered fully. I saw her getting back on a bike—after months of rehab.

A week later I pedaled past the spot where she was hit and tried not to wobble. There were no telltale signs—no skid marks, no bloodstain.

△

In the ER, my imagination first seemed a hindrance, then became a waste of time. Now I realized that imagination unlocked my empathy; it was a key to understanding someone else's suffering. Did I sacrifice my imagination, my empathy, to strengthen my detachment? Mark Epstein writes, "Our humanity resides in our feelings, and we reclaim our humanity when we direct our curiosity at that which we would prefer to avoid."[1]

When advocates got into sticky situations with patients or families, it was usually due to their lack of adequate boundaries or detachment. A lack of boundaries can intrude on patient autonomy—pushing your recommendations, not hearing the "Yes, but." Having an intense emotional reaction to traumas or losing your temper with a family implies a need for some detachment. As a supervisor and coworker, I reminded advocates of the need for both boundaries and detachment. But the third essential concept, unconditional positive regard, was not something I could teach.

I tried to hire for it. I asked for stories of success and failure, of how the interviewee went beyond expectations. I wanted them to share stories that revealed insight into situations and into themselves. I asked what kind of work they *didn't* want to do, what kind of person they found most challenging. I wasn't impressed by denials or insistence that they felt the same toward everyone. If they failed to acknowledge their fears and shortcomings, they were lying—to me and to themselves. If you haven't identified who pushes your buttons and why, your helping is hobbled. Such insight can take years to develop, and for me, required therapy, the study of psychology, and deep reflection. They needed to convince me they had capacity for insight as well as empathy.

Was there ever a time when they cared too much? I also wanted advocate candidates to demonstrate at least an understanding of the need for professional detachment and boundaries. This was something

---

1. Epstein, *The Trauma of Everyday Life*, 97.

easier to model, to instruct on the job, because it could be attached to actions and behavior: We don't give our personal numbers out; we don't befriend a patient or family member; we don't overstep our role, interfering in the work of other staff. Sometimes there are reasons for violating those boundaries, but when that is done unconsciously or habitually, it means you're putting your own needs first.

I began to see that I had constructed boundaries so high, and sowed detachment so wide, that my empathy was hard to reach. I could just look away from the homeless person, from the patient and family that I wasn't being paid to care about, as if caring can be turned on and off easily. There's a balance between self-protection and connection, a dance.

Currently, in retirement, I'm aware of people in my life fighting against the edge of despair. I don't want to join them on that edge, but I do want to feel something, to connect to their emotional experience. That is part of being a member of a family, a good friend, or a community member. This desire to share their pain is something new, or rather, something old reawakened. If I am ready to take on more, then perhaps my mind and heart are no longer overwhelmed. Maybe the barriers are coming down.

△

I am curious about world events, but years ago I switched to print and radio to avoid the relentless images on TV news. My imagination used to provide the pictures. But lately, I've had to seek out those images to feel connected to tragedies befalling strangers. My mind's eye can underestimate the destruction of our wars, the suffering humans inflict on each other and animals, and the damage to our planet.

In 2021, when I'd been retired for a year, my husband and I took a road trip, dodging exposure to Covid, hurricanes and rockslides, blue-green algae, bears seeking human food, and infection-bearing ticks seeking humans as food. We diverted from an interstate traffic jam to wind our way homeward on a country highway that GPS didn't recommend and stubbornly refused to route for us. The reason soon became apparent: We were traveling through an area decimated by a flood.

The demure river now flowing placidly between banks reportedly went rogue when a recent hurricane dumped an astonishing amount of water into it. The water raged, taking homes and vehicles, smothering fields, toppling trees, and drowning people.

We'd heard of this flood. I'd tried to imagine its threat and damage, but even with reports of a dozen or so people missing, my imagination was inadequate. Now we saw how the detritus of lives—clothing, toys, boats—was tossed into treetops and flung onto the newly scoured riverbanks.

Traveling through this community was like being inside a story—a tale I'd heard that seemed far away and long ago. I'd put emotional distance between this flood and my life, my fears of what could happen to my loved ones and me, the same way I thought of accidents, chronic illnesses, and homelessness as other people's problems. I thought I could stay on the periphery, choose when to care. And, I guess to some extent, we all choose when and how much to care. But sometimes, thankfully, our shields of detachment fail.

To be curious about these lives, these disasters, used to seem crude to me. I don't want to consume such scenes as entertainment. Nature can inspire awe in the face of its power as well as relief if you and yours are not hurt by the current disaster. That relief intensifies as natural disasters increase in frequency and proximity.

Turning away from these stories of devastation feels like how I turned away from ER traumas, insulating myself by inattention. Who is protected when I don't connect myself to such stories, employing a "need to know" philosophy? Being curious doesn't mean you care, but if you care, if you want to care, don't you need to be at least a little curious?

△

My lack of curiosity was a protective feature when working, but now that I'm retired, I'm trying to revive it. I find that I'm curious about plenty of things, just not the sensational bits that seem to excite most people. I don't need the gory details of a school shooting; I don't want to see the cars being washed away in a flood, or the victims of a bombing.

One of the easiest ways to stretch my curiosity muscle is with nature. Like many stuck at home during the pandemic, I sought refuge in my backyard, relishing it even more once retired, before our move into an apartment. I spent as much time as I could on our deck overlooking a small patch of grass, anchored by hardwood trees that multiplied beyond the grass and lined a tiny creek.

We had deer, raccoons, opossums, armadillos, coyotes, turtles, snakes, a visit from a fox, and neighborhood cats. But mostly we had birds. I'd come to share my husband's appreciation of birds long ago, but now, in addition to being able to identify a few, I enjoyed just watching them, especially the awkward machinations of the woodpeckers at the bird feeder and the sassy warnings from the wee Carolina wrens.

I regretted not being able to identify all the trees I'd been gazing at for almost three decades. I'd watched some of these trees grow up and others spread out as their companions died and left a space in the canopy.

There are fewer trees where we live now, but the sky is abundant. I watch the transit of clouds and stars. I try to name birds on the wing. When I'm away from my second-story windows, I look closer at what surrounds me. I take seashell books on trips to the ocean, and we use an app to identify wildflowers we find anywhere. There is a sweet pink flower with a yellow center found beside country roads in Virginia and on the dunes of the Outer Banks seashore: the Virginia saltmarsh mallow. I like the way its name tickles my tongue when I say it aloud. The deeper the delight of such discoveries, the further you dive down.

But my mind hasn't fully left the hospital and the staff. In the throes of a pandemic, they were, I knew, exhausted and overwhelmed. We now live only a few blocks away from the hospital, and my thoughts travel there in the scream of a siren or the urgent pulse of a helicopter.

My first thoughts go to the responders. I send a wish for safety to the medics and to the helicopter pilot, who has to negotiate landing in a parking lot close to buildings and in a neighborhood covered by trees. I think of the charge nurse, who I hope received a timely report and has a ready room—nothing stresses a charge nurse like a patient in need with no easy place to put them.

Once the charge nurse knows where she's putting the patient, she assigns the primary nurse, and as this information is typed into the tracking system, it pops up onscreen for the doctors to see. Whoever clicks first gets the patient. I hope that nurse and doctor are rested and ready for this challenge.

I hope there is an advocate to meet the patient and connect them to their family, to ease their time in the ER.

I know that sirens coming from the hospital only mean there *may* be an emergency, but sirens coming toward the hospital have more legitimacy. The medics have confirmed it; now please get out of their way.

When I hear a helicopter, I know it's more likely to be picking up a patient than bringing in one, and that the patient being picked up is most likely a child, because there are children's hospitals a few hours away. I can visualize the flurry of activity that accompanies a helicopter: privacy curtains being drawn near the waiting room entrance to avoid the curious stares of those who have no need to know; nurses and techs standing by for the signal to walk onto the helipad. And I can see the parent summoning courage, standing beside the gurney, ready to go with their sick child or to endure the sight of their child flying away.

So much pain, heartache, fear, and work conveyed by the sounds. I am not curious about the stories. I know it is some variation of someone's luck failing them, or, as some in the ER believe, someone's path intersecting with their fate: "Everything happens for a reason."

△

I am curious about the signs that unhoused persons hold up on street corners and on the downtown sidewalks, but I don't let my eyes linger long enough to read them. I have started meeting their eyes, though. I want them to know they are not invisible—though is it better to be seen by someone who does nothing for you?

I do barely more than nothing. I donate to a shelter monthly and support the food bank. I place dry goods in one of those small open pantries that sprouted up during the pandemic, where anyone can come and take anything. When asked for money, I offer food. Sometimes my offer is accepted and together we walk into a restaurant so I can buy whatever they order.

In the above paragraph, I had originally written an additional line: "And I am glad to do it." But that is not true. In the moment that I am asked for money I notice an undercurrent of anger in myself, and I realize it is always there when I negotiate these interactions. It is resentment for their asking me to stop and take time to hear their request, the unexpected change to my plans. But there's more.

When I feel anger, I know to look deeper for the fear. And there it is: the fear of being physically close to a stranger, fear of harm, fear of being exploited. My fear is part of my defense mode. I am protecting my boundaries, fortifying what I have decided ahead of time I will and will not do. When does a boundary become a barrier?

I'm glad I reach out beyond my fears at such times, but the gesture of one meal feels shamefully inadequate, and my attitude needs work. I also realize that my response violates basic social work principles because I am offering a solution that works for me. I remind myself that helping is complicated.

ER staff are generous in nature but highly suspicious of being conned. In their defense, they are lied to all the time. Lies about medical issues, about social relationships, about habits and addictions, about intentions to follow advice. They are leery of being suckered into the hard luck stories—they've bought into them before only to find that their time and energy was wasted, and, worse, they were made to feel foolish. Their peers ridiculed them for giving extra care to someone taking advantage of their effort.

I didn't care if my extra efforts made me look foolish, at least not when I was in the ER, but out in the world, without the structure of my defined role and my coworkers surrounding me, I am more cautious. I am stingy with my time and attention, and vigilant about my safety. This is not unreasonable, but I would prefer to be less afraid of intrusion, of vulnerability, of connection. I'd like to be more gracious.

Most of my people-related curiosity has turned inward, where it does no one any good, unless you believe that in knowing yourself better you can better help the world. It sounds convenient and self-serving. I want to believe it.

When doing improv skits, actors employ a "Yes, and" method of responding with their partners. They cooperate and stay collaboratively curious to keep the skit rolling. This is against my nature. Instead of *"Yes, and"* my natural response is *"No, because . . ."* My arguments are always at the ready. I am trying to change.

My automatic noes may be a signal of my autonomic nervous system, an instinctive way of reacting in order to feel safe. Making our unconscious reactions conscious is how we start to regulate this system, to keep from overreacting or withdrawing altogether.[2]

For now, I stay curious about my friends and family, widening my circle of concern to include the groups I've become part of since retirement. The only one truly depending on me is my mom. Someday I will offer something of myself to the larger world, but helping people may not be the focus of that offering. Perhaps I have become an antisocial social worker. I'm not sure yet if that's a problem. But I am curious.

Trying to make big-picture differences can seem futile and feels naive, like a little sparrow trying to hold up the sky.

> *It was a chilly, overcast day when the horseman*
> *spied*
> *the little sparrow lying on its back in the middle of*
> *the road.*
> *Reining in his mount he looked down and inquired*
> *of the fragile creature,*
> *"Why are you lying upside down like that?"*

---

2. Dana, *Anchored.*

"I heard the heavens are going to fall today,"
   replied the bird.
The horseman laughed. "And I suppose your spin-
   dly legs can hold up the heavens?"
"One does what one can," said the little sparrow.

—Source unknown

I don't want the heavens to fall on my watch, but when the sky becomes too heavy, the proverbial man on the beach may have the right idea—tossing dying starfish into the surf, one by one. Reconnecting, making a difference, can start with whoever, whatever is in reach, right in front of you.

Rate Yourself in Regard
to Your Humanity

Walking into the farmers market a year before I retired, I saw a tent with a poster asking for volunteers to "complete a survey and get a book." I figured it was a college student's project. I dawdled a moment too long. A man stepped out of the shade of the tent and caught my eye as he walked toward me. Too late I saw the other poster: "Spiritual Survey." I was not looking for a spiritual encounter at the farmers market. At least, not a contrived one.

The man was courteous but gently insistent. He explained that this was part of a global project to better understand the spiritual beliefs of people all over the world. He had a list of questions, including about my faith background and belief in an afterlife. I played my Get Out of Spiritual Awkwardness Free card, telling him I'm an agnostic.

"What exactly does that mean?" he asked.

And before I knew it, I was taking the survey. We came to this question: "Rate yourself (in regard to your humanity) on a scale of 1 to 10 with 10 being perfect."

I had never rated myself as a human before, but immediately assigned myself a seven. I wondered if that was a typical response, or the reflex of a striving-but-stuck Six, full of ambition. I bet most of us believe we are better than average, which isn't statistically possible. I wanted to believe that I'd done more than the average person to earn that higher score, but had I?

Meditation doesn't make you a better person. I read that early on in my mindfulness training and almost quit on the spot. I needed to be a better person—if this wasn't going to make that happen, then what was the point? I decided the person who wrote that didn't want or need improving as badly as I did. Or maybe they weren't doing it right.

A poet friend told me that my poems reflect my desire for self-improvement. That seems like the worst poetic legacy ever. It's embarrassing. My need to be better, to do better, seems to leak into everything.

If you sit on the cushion often enough and become aware of your thoughts, you have a shot at sustaining some of that awareness off the cushion. You begin to see how immediate your response is to certain triggers, like you've programmed yourself, and during those emotional moments, you may find you have a space you didn't have before—a pause before you react—and in that pause lies a choice. Maybe you don't have to curse the driver that cut you off, the persistent salesperson on the phone, or your husband, who clearly wasn't listening to you.

You can continue reacting, overreacting, defending, and attacking, or you can try something different. Choosing to do something different, to *be* different, could mean that you step closer to whatever is your definition of a better person.

I once took a complaint from a patient we saw for a mental health crisis. She felt our staff needed more training in dealing with patients like her, because while she was responding emotionally due to the stress of her ailment, she felt our staff reacted emotionally as well: "But you! You reacted back!" I understood what she meant, and it was more than a fair point.

She was the one experiencing the crisis; we were the professionals at our place of work, with our team, essentially in our home. She was the one having the bad day, the worst-case scenario. She expected more from us.

Being able to slow that automatic emotional reaction to someone else's emotional intensity is one benefit of meditation. I first enrolled in a mindfulness stress-reduction meditation course when my dad was diagnosed with terminal pancreatic cancer. This disease moves quickly and has few treatment options in the late stages. Dad chose hospice care as soon as he was diagnosed, which meant he would die at home, with my mother providing the majority of his care.

I was permitted to work four-day weeks so I could make the four-hour trip to their home on Fridays and return on Mondays. The main way I helped was by sleeping in the room next to Dad to assist him at night so that Mom could sleep.

I brought them food, watched old shows with my dad, and joined in on meetings with hospice workers. I took long walks alone on the golf course at night, my dad wistfully remarking that he'd give anything to go with me. But he was in a wheelchair by then.

I knew this experience would be hard enough without my devolving into old patterns—immature reactions to old provocations. (Do we all become twelve again when we go home?) I wanted my visits to make things better, not worse. Prior years in therapy had taken me a long way toward understanding my family dynamics and myself, but I looked to meditation to change my response in the moment.

During the day I was on my laptop too much, a way to have time to myself, to distance myself from the intimacy of dying—an intimacy I could more easily tolerate with strangers than my parents. I didn't become the very best version of myself, but I was physically there and as emotionally present as I could be. Perhaps I was "good enough."

My dad was unconscious his last night and died while I sat beside him. I woke my mom and aunt and we all said goodbye to him. Mom called the hospice nurse. I made a pot of coffee, then trudged to a back bedroom. I texted my husband and asked him to tell our kids. I didn't want to talk to anyone; I wanted to sleep.

Mom later said she was touched by the gentleness of the hospice nurse as she washed his body and prepared him for the funeral home. A neighbor told us that she was walking her dog early that morning when she saw the hearse and snapped to attention, holding a salute. I missed my dad and I hated what he'd gone through, but I never cried.

Three years later, when my mom moved to our town and I became her caregiver, I went back for more mindfulness training. I needed to move the needle further, to become a better person and a better daughter—*stat.*

△

After steadily winnowing my time and tasks down to the least amount possible that could still justify my being on the payroll, I finally opted to retire. Working fewer hours had brought me greater life satisfaction, but the work was less satisfying. After all the times I nearly walked out in protest, in a bold stand for a principle or a patient, when it came time to go, I went out with a whisper. I was too removed from the patients' experience and too disconnected from ER operations to have an impact, to influence change. I could help the hospital by encouraging patients to follow up or by smoothing over their complaints, but that did not meet my need for making a difference in individual lives.

I retired in February 2020. Our town locked down in March. I couldn't know that the timing would happen this way, but I'd been expecting a pandemic ever since avian flu threatened to cross the ocean years ago, when I was sent to a meeting for pandemic planning.

Every couple of years, when a disease mounted an attack on the world (such as avian flu, Ebola, SARS, or the Zika virus), I thought, *This could be The One.* I didn't predict Covid—I would never have guessed how thoroughly it impacted us—but I was not surprised that we were finally experiencing a global pandemic.

If you believe that things happen for a reason, then you may believe I was fated to retire right before Covid. But that logic implies there's a reason for all my coworkers not to be spared that experience—a reason that I got a loving universe, and they did not.

△

At the farmers market, taking that spiritual survey, I mentally defended my better-than-average humanity rating with my choice to be a social worker. But although I have spent my life in jobs that are expressly about helping others, I have not done so with a pure heart—to paraphrase the Book of Common Prayer, part of my old Episcopal "faith background."

I was paid to help people.

"We have not loved our neighbors as ourselves," continues the confession. I flick off my helper mode as though it's a taxicab light. When I clocked out each day, that light went off. You want my help? Wait 'til my light is back on. I'm compartmentalizing here, people. It's a coping mechanism. Look it up.

Though I manage to mostly be a helpful, friendly sort of person, I don't go much out of my way for a stranger. Still, I rated myself as a seven.

We moved on to the next survey question: "If you were at the gates of heaven, what would you say to try to get in?"

My reply: "I wasn't perfect, but I did try, and I did care."

With all respect to the paving crew on that road to hell, I still believe that efforts and intentions count for something if they're sincere and not limited to couch potato philosophizing. Yet I feel guilty. I know I am not all I could be in regard to my humanity. I wonder if whoever wrote this survey expected these answers to inspire guilt to motivate church attendance. But my guilt isn't limited to the needs of mankind—it extends to the entire Earth and beyond. Where's the church for that? How do we atone for "what we have done and what we have left undone"?

The survey ended, and the man told me that I gave exceptional answers and was generous with my time. He told me about their church and invited me to attend.

He did not offer a book, and I did not ask. What would a real Seven have done?

△

Erikson's final stage of adult development—Integrity vs. Despair— challenges the healthy individual to find meaning in their lives, to figure out what it means to have lived so that they can face death. Failure to meet this challenge results in despair. No one wants to go out like that.

The stage starts at age sixty-five and ends when you die. I've jumped the gun on this one. I like having a head start because we can't know how long we'll live. I know that the worst can and does happen—like Covid.

Some speak of gifts from the pandemic. Most do this in a whisper because they know they are lucky. None of us were spared the stress and the new limits to our old world. But some of us didn't have to school our children, or wear a mask through a twelve-hour shift while dealing with unruly customers or critically ill patients. Some of us didn't have to leave our aged parent isolated in a facility. We didn't lose a loved one to the virus or get seriously ill ourselves.

The onset of Covid was harsh and terrifying, but it also slowed down time and withdrew the usual distractions. For me, being newly retired when Covid hit, I could stay home, focusing on the task at hand: downsizing to move out of our house and into an in-town apartment.

The house we were leaving was the one we built one year after I started at the ER. I'd had the job and the house for over twenty-eight years. Now I'd left the job, and the two of us were about to leave the house.

Day after day I sifted through memorabilia I'd tucked into box after box over the years: photos, certificates, letters, children's artwork. I took a break in the afternoon with the same walk around the neighborhood I'd been taking for almost three decades. I read about "clinging" from the Buddhist perspective—holding something too tightly evokes suffering because everything changes. I could keep a few things, but most objects had to go. I texted pictures of the kids' artwork to them, I composed poems about sorting through life's detritus, I wrote an essay about keeping my daughter's blue hoodie hanging in my closet. I hugged my son's teddy bear, tucking her into a box to keep, and I found appreciative homes for many books.

I loved this house, these trees, the wildlife passing through. I cherished the gift of being in a place long enough to see how its landscape changed—something my peripatetic childhood had denied me.

In quitting my job, I'd already lost a huge part of my identity. How could I let go of this home that was such an emotional anchor? I realized that I didn't have to stop loving it to let it go. It comforted me to know that it would continue to exist, in reality and in my mind and heart; I just would no longer get to live there.

Still, I needed more than self-help books and my journal to accept all this change and uncertainty. When Covid hit, the local meditation group, which I'd never found time for, put their weekly sessions online. I now had the time. I learned to Zoom.

The doer in me takes pride in having managed retirement and a move during Covid. But the bigger accomplishment was establishing a meditation practice, going from *doing* toward *being*. The meditation group had both new and experienced meditators, and my practice grew with their support. Still wobbly in my skills, I nevertheless took turns leading meditation. This was a group where we learned from each other, and that learning was often experiential. Doing was a necessary part of it, but it was in the service of being, and that made a shift inside me. Hence Covid's gift to me—a world swept clean of diverting busyness. My life made sparse and the present moment revealed.

Until this quieter, slower time, I had continued to compartmentalize. I believed it was a key component in keeping my sanity. As if I could toggle seamlessly between work mode and non-work mode, social worker me and creative me, Mom me and Boss me. Like so many of my tools for surviving the ER, compartmentalization came with a cost: a barrier to a richer experience of life. The task at hand deserves your focus, but if you shut down parts of yourself to do that task, how will you ever become whole again?

Mindfulness practice endorses a more holistic approach. I agreed in principle, but in my early practice I regarded *being* as just another mode. I stayed in motion until the second I sat on the cushion and changed the channel, attempting mindfulness in whatever sliver of time I had scheduled for contemplative mode.

Then a different sort of book snuck under my radar and tripped the fuse for my compartmentalization wiring. David Abram's *Becoming Animal* describes how he experiences nature. He seems to drop down into it, advocating "a way of thinking enacted as much by the body as by the mind, informed by the humid air and the soil and the quality of our breathing, by the intensity of our contact with the other bodies that surround."[1]

This was a reminder that a key to slowing down the brain that plans and the body that acts was to sink into awareness of our senses. I loved my nature walks and observing wildlife wherever I found it. How would it be if I were less the outside observer and more a part of the landscape? Sitting long enough to feel part of the woods, being still enough that birds and deer would forage around me. I eased into a different attitude, staying aware of the traps of trying too hard and of having rigid expectations about "performance," attachment to the kind of experience I wanted to have.

I could take my meditation off the cushion, but only if I loosened the bindings and blurred the labels that placed my experiences into categories on the day's schedule. Instead of flipping a switch, I tried leaving the light on.

△

When I took that survey at the farmers market, I was still working for the ER. I wondered if once I retired I would feel a stronger compulsion to help people—when I'm no longer paid to care, will I care more?

The jury's still out. I catch myself doing small things in secret, as if I'm that off-duty cabbie picking up hitchhikers in her own car. Is that being a good human or is it just habit?

A new acquaintance, Jackie, gave me a chance to do more for someone in need, but I blew it. She'd crossed paths with a woman living in her car. Jackie gave her money and information about shelters, but the woman had already tried those resources. Later, Jackie came up with a new plan to help the woman but couldn't find her. The car had been parked near our new apartment—would I look for her to give her Jackie's phone number?

Yes, of course. I combined my searches with trips to the mailbox and dumpsters. I texted my lack of success and added that I would

---

1. David Abram, *Becoming Animal* (Vintage Books, 2011), 4.

expand my walks and "keep an eye out." Jackie suggested that I search first thing in the morning if I was up. I am usually up early, but if the day is a success, I'm not dressed until noon. A younger woman might throw a hoodie over her pajama bottoms and walk the block, but my generation doesn't travel far in their pajamas—maybe onto the front porch or down the driveway to get the paper, the distance determined by the number of seconds it would take to scoot inside if spotted.

I don't know if Jackie knew I was once a social worker, that I am trying to recover from identity enmeshment. But what does that mean? That I'm trying to not care as much? Jackie probably expected me to make a more concerted effort, possibly overestimating my need to help and my sense of social obligation.

In social work practice we are warned not to make a bigger effort than the client makes. I have perverted this maxim to relieve myself of big gestures, like getting dressed and leaving my home much earlier than planned. Of course, the woman living in her car didn't know I was trying to find her, and I didn't know what kind of effort she was making.

I feel the need to defend myself. Experienced social workers have been "Yes, but"-ed many times. We know that even people with intense needs prefer their own solutions. But we also know that people get desperate, and sometimes what you're offering is exactly what they need or comes close enough. I am trying to cut through my layers of jaded rationalizations to say I still believe a caring person can make a difference; I am just skeptical of the methods. Still, trying any way that you can is admirable.

I did not find the woman. If I were a better person, I'd have gotten dressed earlier. In trying to avoid resentment (my own), I've created a pile of remorse and stepped right into it.

Reaching for redemption, I broke my rule about never giving money, when I encountered a family with young children. The father held a sign up asking for rent money. A new rental agency had taken over several properties in our town. Rents were raised significantly, and government housing vouchers were no longer accepted. Many people were evicted or soon would be. I had to walk right beside the man with his toddler. I tried to give him information about a local agency that helps with rent, but there was a language barrier. I handed him cash, nodding at the whispered thanks from his young wife, who was holding a baby. I got home and emailed a friend who works at the agency that gives rent assistance, and later that day she replied with a resource that is well equipped to help Spanish speakers. I wrote the number down and went looking for the family, but they were gone. I put that number in my car, but I've never seen them again.

A month later, as I pulled into a parking space at a drugstore, a man stood a few feet away and raised a hand to get my attention. I have been approached in parking lots before. It feels threatening. Parking lot solicitations evoke my most aggressive refusals. But this man kept his distance. I stayed in the car and rolled down the window. He had a long story and started by telling me his name. I was impatient, wanting to say, *"Just make the ask."* But I listened.

He held up documentation of his stay in a local hotel room. He would get paid tomorrow, but the hotel was kicking him and his wife out today unless they came up with thirty-four dollars. I had two twenties in my wallet. My mind swirled with options: Just give him the name of the agency where my friend works, or give him twenty dollars and the name of the agency. I told myself I was not obligated to completely solve his problem. But then I recalled my remorse from the other two situations.

I rolled up the window, and he stepped back. I got out the money and opened the door. I stepped forward and handed him the two twenties. He stammered a thanks and held up a card for a free burrito—an exchange of offerings. Don't I want it? "No, thanks. Good luck to you." I locked my car and walked into the store.

I broke my rules. I felt slightly better. If his story was true, then I made a difference, at least for one night. And if his story wasn't true? I realized that I don't care much about that anymore. What bothers me now is that I didn't give him the resource information. He's probably going to need it, and to just hand him cash and turn on my heel feels dismissive. But I wanted our awkward interaction to end as quickly as possible for us both.

Feeling better about myself is apparently entwined with believing that I am helping others. This is an old discovery dusted off for my new reality. Time and attention invite connection but carry risk. Maybe I need new rules or no rules at all.

My Meaning-Making Machinery

Humans are pattern-seeking creatures. We sift through life's minutiae for signs that indicate meaning behind life-changing events. The need to understand the why about what happens to us here and beyond led me from a belief in a standard Christian afterlife to a belief in reincarnation, then to a certainty of uncertainty. This sequence seems less like evolution than devolution, like going from a floor plan to a nebula.

I stayed in the reincarnation stage a long while. When I was twelve, my favorite aunt gave me a copy of *Be Here Now* by Ram Dass, which served as my gateway to alternative thinking. So many things appealed to me in the reincarnation paradigm: a sense of justice, an economy of resources (recycling souls), a way to extend learning opportunities, an explanation for dreams and déjà vu. But ultimately the logistics exhausted me.

I shifted to agnosticism. I can allow all possibilities with no obligation to understand the details. For me, agnosticism says, "Life is a mystery that we need not bother even trying to figure out." This has freed up a lot of time.

I was still in my reincarnation phase when I got the job in the ER, and it played well with "things happen for a reason." But while some people can sustain a belief in a logical universe while working in the ER, I could not.

I went into free fall. If nothing happened for a reason, could anything happen to anybody at any time? Check. Trauma forces one to face the random nature of reality. In *The Trauma of Everyday Life*, Epstein writes of the deep divide between the reality of the person who experiences trauma and the reality of nearly everyone else. He says this chasm deepens the trauma because communication about it is impossible.

I don't blame the ER for making me face the realities of our mortality. Anyone paying attention to the world around them is presented with the same challenge: how to cobble together meaning in our lives and in the world despite our harsh experience—Integrity vs. Despair, Erikson's final stage.

If you can make your tight belief system jump through life's hoops, you may have a softer landing when the rug comes out from under you. Believing in a plan, or a system of checks and balances, has to be better than the utter bewilderment of concluding that life's ups and downs are the luck of the draw. You may recall that I've never considered myself lucky. ("Heads or tails?") If I believe I have little power to limit my future suffering, then all I have is the present. This doesn't mean that I live in a hedonistic way, or that I stop doing reasonable things for my future health and happiness or to help others and the planet. But I want to shift my attention to what I can control, to being in the present moment.

Fear of death, my own and of those I love, is a constant challenge. The thought of those I love most leaving me stirs up both the ache of anticipated loss and a yearning to have them close always. But nothing stays the same. And what happens to me when I die? Where does this love of life and learning and nature go when my heart stops? If there's no heaven or reincarnation, what happens? And if the answer is "nothing," how do I manage the terror of that abyss?

The comedian Ricky Gervais speaks openly about his belief that when the body dies, we are completely gone. He says it doesn't worry him because nothingness is nothing, like being sedated during surgery—you just turn off. He says the hard part is now, the worry of it. But he doesn't seem worried. I marvel that someone so successful could have so little ego, or an ego mature enough to not get tangled up in thoughts of obliteration. My ego has miles to go.

If I hadn't worked in the ER, I believe this crisis would have been postponed. I would have moved through years free from the burden of knowing that death's visits are ill-timed, random, and inexplicable. In the land of worst-case scenarios, you see that people depart unexpectedly all the time, which makes the unexpected expected—we are surprised by nothing.

$$\triangle$$

Recently my husband and I were biking in a forested area and got caught in a sudden thunderstorm. The lightning popped all around us. We were an hour from our car, and there was no shelter any closer. My instinct was to keep riding—faster. But I don't ride very fast, and we'd been going hard for more than two hours. I reached a fork in the trail, where I found my husband waiting by his bike.

My husband asked, "Do we stand together, or do we stand apart?" I fully understood what he didn't say. Our thoughts went to the same place—our children. They were adults now, out of college. We no longer had to split the odds.

"Together," I said. It was a perverse feeling of peace, perhaps because it was new: For the first time in our married lives, we could opt to die together.

I don't know if standing still in a forest during lightning is safer than frantically biking through it. But once I subdued my flight instinct, it felt better to stand and face it. We stood side by side in the rain, glimpsing an angry sky between the waving arms of tree branches, willing our ears to discern cracks of electrical bolts from cracks of exploding wood, hoping if a tree fell, we could dodge it. The storm soon passed, and we rode out together.

I feel the closest to dying when I fly. I never assume I will survive a trip. I try to tie up loose ends before leaving. Once before flying, I emailed a project to a friend *in case anything happens*, so attached was I to my life and my ambitions, so under the thrall of my dramatic imagination, so desperate for something of me to endure.

My mom tells me that my dad would purchase catastrophic insurance on any of us when we flew—and he was a pilot. Once, when I was on a flight without my husband, my teenage children argued over who had to sit next to me. My daughter lost. When our plane shook with turbulence from a storm that required us to make three attempts to land, I shook, I gasped, I clutched her hand, I yearned for solid ground. My daughter became the adult, reassuring me, admitting that it was rough and scary, then saying with some amusement, "But it's not like we're gonna die." My eyes widened in challenge. This seemed exactly how death on an airplane could play out. She scoffed, recounting statistics and the experience and skills of our crew. Mere facts couldn't allay my terror, but she believed in those facts, and I believed in her. And that helped. It also helps to watch the crew. They keep their invisible masks of calm securely in place. I know they are wearing masks, but it still helps.

What throws me is the apparent ease of the passengers. Surely I'm not the biggest scaredy-cat in a plane full of regular people. Despite a few phobias, I never thought of myself as a fearful person. As a child, I was somewhat of a daredevil with my horse; as a teen I got certified as a scuba diver. Some would say my decision to have my children born at home was brave. I've kayaked in white-water rivers. And, despite that lightning storm, bear and rattlesnake sightings, and a few hard crashes, I still love to mountain bike on challenging trails deep in a forest, sometimes alone. But even on a rough flight, no one else seems to be at risk of freaking out.

I tell myself the other passengers are braver, better actors, repressive types, or taking drugs. Maybe those passengers are smarter, have less imagination, are less emotional, or are able to put their trust in facts, as my daughter did. Maybe they've dissected the horror of their mortality, constructed some meaning of life and death that brings them peace. I am jealous. Most likely they haven't worked for years in a place where someone dies nearly every day.

Once my kids became adults, these fears shifted. I was no longer ruled by an instinctive mandate to keep them alive, and a bonus gift was that my own mortality didn't matter so much. My fear of flying, now that I was free of the weight of responsibility, was tamped down to anxious discomfort.

△

Meanwhile the fear while driving got worse. My daily life became more complicated by drive-arounds from my trigger spots. My comfort with risk is proportional to my belief in the amount of control I think I have and my perceived confidence in my skills. But anxiety has nothing to do with the reality of skills, and having chronic anxiety means calling on your courage constantly. Recalling that these concerns were dismissed the last time I asked a medical provider about anxiety medication, and still reluctant to see a therapist, I redoubled my efforts to cure myself.

In my early fifties, when submitting a short story to an alternative zine, I saw a listing of their publications, including a tiny book on anxiety. I bought it. The book, titled *This Is Your Brain on Anxiety*, takes pains to appeal to younger readers, but I still felt included in its basic, conversational approach, which reassured me I wasn't alone.[1]

I learned to recognize and rate my attacks. Giving your anxiety a name is suggested. I went with Heffalump—the elusive creature of the Hundred Acre Wood that Winnie-the-Pooh fears, who turns out to be adorable and harmless (unless you have honey). Heffalumps are a symbol of imagination, overgrown to the size of an elephant. Perhaps imagination could be part of the cure as well as the cause.

A meditation practice is tremendously helpful with anxiety. The little book espoused meditation principles, breathing deeply, recognizing those panicky moments rather than trying to ignore them or push them away. I learned to breathe my way through those times and reduce my heart palpitations and crazy-making thoughts. I began manufacturing fewer incidents in general.

I was open to learning new coping strategies and avoiding medication. I figured I just had to get myself through a few more years until I could retire, and then all the stress would melt away. But that assumes

---

1. Faith Harper, *This Is Your Brain on Anxiety: What Happens and What Helps* (Microcosm Publishing, 2018).

anxiety follows logic. My neurological wiring was jacked up (a medical term) with well-worn pathways designed for delivery of panic.

I retired the month before we locked down for Covid, at age fifty-seven. My mother's husband (she remarried at age eighty-two) became terminally ill, and I stepped into a more active caregiving role with the ever-present fear of getting and spreading Covid to them, who were among the most vulnerable to Covid. Also at this time was the move my husband and I made from a house in a subdivision to an apartment in the city. Covid, caregiving, and moving—retirement was not turning out to be as relaxing as I had expected. Did any of this matter? I don't know. I just know the anxiety wasn't noticeably better after retirement.

A year into retirement, and about fifteen years after that talk with the nurse practitioner, my new primary doctor apologized that she had to screen me for mental health issues. Caught off guard, I was honest. She asked detailed questions and encouraged me to try medication. After reading about possible side effects and polling friends for their advice and experience, I tried it. The medication is helping. I can once again drive into Atlanta and anywhere I want, with only the rational fear of knowing that driving is the most dangerous thing we do.

Anxiety can be debilitating. What level of discomfort can be tolerated versus what's too disruptive is an individual calculation. I have no doubt that leaving the ER benefited my mental health, but how would I be now if I had never worked there, and is it too late to reverse the corruption in my wiring?

△

I still haven't reconciled with the idea of nonexistence, but it's one of those things I am comfortable being uncomfortable about. Recently I've been thinking about the experience of "flow state," those moments when we lose ourselves. This term is often used in regard to an activity, such as when an athlete or performer is completely in sync with their endeavor, but I like to think of flow state as the river we come from and will one day return to. Alison Bechdel paraphrases Zen master

Shunryu Suzuki as saying, "Before we're born, we're like the river up above. Then we're separated from that oneness into droplets. We forget that we're part of the river, and we feel fear. But soon enough we join the river again."[2]

Most days I take the prospect of oblivion in stride, pretty sure that, at a minimum, the end brings peace. On my best days (or, rather, minutes), I am in the Now, appreciating the moment without existential dread—unless that moment is on an airplane.

Separate from fear and faith and fate is the matter of synchronicity: the idea that coincidences matter, whether it's the way new information seems to drop out of the ethosphere and into our lives—the poem or book that acts as the perfect salve for a new ache or question—or the way a chance meeting turns into a lifelong friendship. If you believe in synchronicity, then you will recognize odd bits about being human not as random edges to our experiences but as potential signposts: Turn here, explore this, join up. I used to embrace this notion, but when I tossed out "things happen for a reason," I gave synchronicity the boot as well.

Although they seem related, I now see them differently. In "things happen for a reason," the belief is in a universe with a specific plan for each of us. (Or did you think it was only for you?) Synchronicity seems to me to be almost the opposite—not a blueprint but an invitation.

I don't think the universe has a specific plan for me. But I have a sort of specific plan for me, and I would like the universe's help. I haven't completely abandoned the idea of a Source in our universe. And in my universe that Source is benevolent, though mysteriously negligent.

When synchronicity feels too New Agey for me, I remember that the term was coined by Carl Jung. In discussions about synchronicity, he shares a story from a session he had with a woman he describes as highly educated and rational. He recognized the challenge of getting her to move past her rationalizations and work at a deeper level. He wrote of his yearning for something "unexpected and irrational" to break through her intellectualism. While listening to her describe

---

2. Alison Bechdel, *The Secret to Superhuman Strength* (Mariner Books, 2021).

a dream in which she was given a piece of jewelry, a golden scarab, he heard a tapping at the window. He saw a large colorful insect. He opened the window and caught it in his hand. "It was a scarabaeid beetle, or common rose-chafer (*Cetonia aurata*), whose gold-green colour most nearly resembles that of a golden scarab. I handed the beetle to my patient with the words, 'Here is your scarab.'" This synchronous experience "broke the ice of her intellectual resistance."[3]

△

I've calibrated my meaning-making machinery to reach an obvious conclusion: My life means what I make of it. I don't turn over the meaning-making to a specific belief system or to spiritual leaders, though I do value their teachings. Coincidences have to pretty much knock me down to get my attention. But when they do, I try to see them as seeds of potential. I consider if I want them to germinate. What grows can be fascinating—the confluence of present time on this body and mind, manifesting into a tangible music, the soundtrack of my life.

Early on in writing this book, I struggled for a way to fold in social work practice guidelines, Erikson's theories, Jung's psychology, Campbell's hero myths, and Josselson's studies of feminine identity. They seemed too disparate to put together, yet taking one without the others was like wedging my experiences into a too-tight corset, denying the expansive breadth of my experience.

After months of reading and reviewing materials and grasping for insight into how to include them, I had this dream:

> *I am in the administrative office area of the ER, which,*
> *in my last years, was in the basement. It is after hours. I*

3. Carl G. Jung, "Synchronicity: An Acausal Connecting Principle." R. F. C. Hull, Trans. In H. Read, M. Fordham, & G. Adler, Eds., *The Collected Works of C. G. Jung, Volume 8.* (Princeton University Press, 1973), para 843, 982. Retrieved November 8, 2022, from http://naqiao.hk/libros_fortea/synchronicity_an_acausal_connecting_principlp-CG_Jung.pdf.

am finally quitting for the day and passing through the main office area. All the cubicles are empty. The light is very dim and reddish, like night-vision lighting. I come upon two women standing outside of the locked door of the ER director's office. I know that they are a film crew, here working on some project. They are glad to see me—everyone else has gone home. One is the film's director, and the other is the cinematographer; she holds her tripod.

My boss wanted them to write out the project for her. They have done this, and the film director holds a stack of small but thick books with red covers edged in gold. I tell them I am the only one here, but I can get the books to my boss. I will put them in my office. The three of us step toward my door.

I take out my key and open my office, which is much bigger than it was in waking reality. It is dark inside, lit only by lamps on their lowest setting. I take the stack of books and walk to my desk. The director and cinematographer stand by the door, unsure if they should come in, looking down at the floor, where there are large sheets of drawing paper.

I explain that the artwork on the floor is from an artist who needed me to keep it there for her. We all realize that I am now keeping safe yet another woman's art. In taking the books, my office seems to become a sort of repository of feminine creative expression.

We gaze at the artwork on the floor. It is made up of pieces of paper painted with swirling designs in rich colors. The artist has written on the underside of each paper—that side is down. I lift one to show them. This artwork is over the entire floor like giant stepping stones.

I take one of the red books from the stack the film director gave me. I tell her I want to read it myself; I am interested in her project. She says that she'd love to "have a real writer's take on it." She means me! She knows I am a writer even though that is not my job in this place. I feel seen. I am pleased and eager to know more about her vision for her project.

I awoke from the dream in a fragile state, at risk of being crushed by my waking brain, eager to seize the day's activities. If I had jumped out of bed, it would have disappeared, never to be fully known. Lying still helps to anchor dreams. It's like listening in person to an orchestra playing. Long after the last notes, the vibration and resonance continue. I felt the tingling of a connection, an unexpected encounter. I let it soak in, yet put it aside.

We tend to dismiss our dreams. Even after years of keeping a dream journal, I have to convince myself that a dream is worth writing down. Perhaps because I've kept a dream journal, I have become a dream snob—making hasty judgments about which get written down and considered and which get fed into the shredder of "I don't need to remember this."

It's handy, this neural mechanism I assume exists to declutter our mental storage space, releasing that which our ego decides we don't need to keep. But thankfully a dream sometimes holds on tenaciously, its fingertips grasping, resisting the blades of that shredder. If you're paying attention, you pull those dreams back and reconnect with the feeling the dream imparted.

Some dreams have a persistent echo that calls for days until finally I override my dismissing ego and look more closely. I always find something worth my attention. I am still learning to listen.

This dream barely survived. I pulled it back from the shredder but didn't write it down and ponder it fully until days later. If you're not buying this dream stuff, then these stakes are anticlimactic, whereas for me it's an "all was almost lost" plot point. I almost destroyed something that I've decided was essential in my struggle with the biggest writing project of my life.

Yes, I've *decided.* I don't assume the dream objectively, empirically, means anything. Without me here to prop it up, to make the dream tangible to my waking self and apply personal meaning, it would just evaporate. I'm not using this dream to generalize about our brains and the world around them, or imply a link to an esoteric nature of the universe. My dream means something only because it means something to *me*.

We are, all of us, trying to make meaning of our existence. A constant search for signs that reverberate with individualized meaning is too saturated with a "me" orientation for my taste. I'm not signing up for "everything means anything you want it to mean," but much in life is beyond concrete objectivity, and we can't escape our compulsion to make meaning even if we want to. Perhaps my efforts are no different from the superstitions held by ER staff, and I'm sorry now if I ridiculed them.

I understand why their beliefs work for them, and I have found a mechanism that works for me. I confine such inspiration to my own body—the dreams, intuitions, interactions, observations, and sensory input that I experience. I don't believe that the universe is intimately involved in my life, but I want to be intimately involved with the universe. I believe there is a connection between me and everything else. Not because I'm special, but because of the exact opposite.

Being human doesn't extract us from the network of nature, but it can blind us to it. Our brains tell us we are above it, separate. But I am a creature, a living thing, connected to other living things in ways we don't fully understand but which I believe exist. If I don't constantly dismiss and belittle that connection, I may glean a clue from it now and then. And even if all this is a big bunch of hooey, it is at least an interesting way to live.

Reflecting on this dream later, I scolded my dream-self for my dream actions, or lack thereof. Maybe that film director's book held the key to the structure I was looking for! Why didn't my dream-self crack open that book as soon as she gave it to me? But if I had, could I have read the words?

Through a Gestalt therapy group in college, I learned to interpret my dreams by considering each element potentially representative of an aspect of myself. I do not limit myself to this framework, but with this dream it was helpful to consider one aspect within myself as a cinematographer, able to make my work vivid and visceral. There is a director aspect who has a vision guiding the project; there is an unseen boss, arbitrating value and risk; and there is an unseen, unknown artist who is creating outside of the frames of the scene, whose work has gotten only as far as the floor of my office, though it nevertheless lies there respected. The me in waking life is represented by the social worker who is unable to leave the office until she ensures the work of these women is safe.

This dream did not yield a road map for this book, but it gave me the encouragement I needed. To me it meant that I had the key to unlock these artistic expressions, to make those connections. I still didn't know how, but I believed it was possible. I felt the support and guidance of those other women artists—other aspects of my Self. "The core of the dream is not the manifest content but the emotional experience."[4] In locking away my ER experiences from the rest of my life, I failed to incorporate them into my awareness. Writing this book was my key to integrating my ER experience. On the floor are the stepping stones of "what happened." I could just walk on top of them, or I could flip them over to see what is written underneath.

Glinda the Good Witch didn't tell Dorothy how to leave Oz for home. The answer was inside Dorothy all along. Those unseen words in the red books in my dream are a wisdom for me to discover. My subconscious self provided the dream images; now it's up to my conscious self to make of them what I will, to manifest them in the waking world.

I hold the key to that dream office full of creative expression: "Here is your scarab."

---

4. Michael Egan, quoted in Epstein, *The Trauma of Everyday Life*, 93.

The Return

The hero's return is the last part of the story in Joseph Campbell's hero's journey framework. The journey began with a call to adventure, met with trepidation or overconfidence. I had a bit of both. Happy in my adoption job, I just needed a way to earn more money and get insurance. I wasn't looking for excitement, but the challenge of medical social work intrigued me, and I felt certain I could do the job despite my issues with fainting at the sight or mention of blood.

If we were watching this as a movie, this is when we'd shout at the screen, *"No! Don't do it!"* But the hero has to go on the adventure, or there isn't a story. They don't always know it's going to be an adventure, much less a life-changing one; they're just traveling somewhere new, learning a new skill, meeting their soulmate, or taking a part-time job.

The hero answers the call. Along the way I made friends and then lost most of them, faced villains, and got tangled in a spell of delusion that made me forget I was not in the real world but in the land of worst-case scenarios. Twenty-nine years later, when I took the path out, the difference in my exterior life was immediate. My days were no longer full of the stories of strangers. I no longer had to listen deeply to tales of pain and hardship, or feel responsible for making a difference. I was far away from the sadness and intensity of the ER, but my body acted as if it were still in there, in that place of trauma and death, sickness and hopelessness.

The hero does not return empty-handed. She is expected to bring home treasure. The treasure may be intangible, only wisdom to show for her trials, but I felt no wiser, and so, answered another call to adventure.

I traveled back to my time in the ER, to understand how and why it changed me. I wondered if this journey of discovery would help me change back, to the caring, connected person I once was. But there is no going back to the old me. Writing this book was another turn on the spiral, my golden elixir revealed in the remembered values of imagination, curiosity, and listening—my paths to caring and connection, not just to others but to myself.

The return home is a return to ourselves. In *Women Who Run with the Wolves*, Dr. Clarissa Pinkola Estés also attributes the delay of the return to a woman's "overidentification with the healer archetype," an ideal that functions as a trap for many women. It's a compulsion to "heal everything, fix everything . . . introduced into our psyches when we are very young." She goes on: "The exact answer to 'Where is home?' is more complex . . . but in some way it is an internal place, a place somewhere in time rather than space, where a woman feels of one piece."[1]

Connecting to myself meant listening and learning from my body as well as my mind. A close friend recommended the book *Anchored: How to Befriend Your Nervous System Using Polyvagal Theory*. The author, Deb Dana, explores how we are impacted by our autonomic nervous system, the system which regulates our breathing, heart rate, and digestion, without any attention from us.

"Vagal refers to the vagus nerve, which in fact is not a single nerve but rather a bundle of nerves that begins in the brainstem and travels through the body."[2] The polyvagal theory suggests that we have evolved three ways of responding to stimulation. These building blocks came into being one after the other, with one hundred million or so years between each, with each new system "joining the older system instead of replacing it."

1. Clarissa Pinkola Estés, *Women Who Run with the Wolves* (Ballantine Books, 1996), 282–283.
2. Dana, *Anchored*.

Newest on the scene is the ventral vagal: a system of connection, a positive way to adapt to life and connect to others—going with the flow. Older is our system of action, called the sympathetic, which includes our fight-or-flight reactions to stress. And older still is the dorsal vagal, a system of withdrawal, which can mean disconnection, physical immobilization, and emotional shutdown.

If the sympathetic or dorsal system dominates, your nervous system may need retuning, a means to persuade it that you are not in danger. Of course, if you are in frequent danger, then your nervous system is doing its job. I am not in constant danger; my nervous system is just scrambled.

Therapies working with the polyvagal theory focus on connection to body sensations and safe connection to others. Awareness of what's happening inside your body with your breath, heartbeat, and muscle tension helps you understand how your body is perceiving safety or danger in the present moment. Although we can learn to self-regulate, Dana states that our need to connect to others is ongoing and "the foundation for navigating daily living." This co-regulation is why talking to a friend helps us when we're stressed—we need others to turn to who themselves are regulated.

The impact of traumatic events is recognized by Dana, but she assures us we can enhance our ability to cope by recognizing our physiological responses and seeking the comfort of those who help us regulate.

This theory helps me understand the significant differences in individuals' responses to similar experiences—why some of us are more resilient than others. It also explains why loneliness is so detrimental: Our need for each other is baked in.

Another way I work on connection with my body is through massage therapy. In my early thirties, having previously considered bodywork just an occasional indulgence, I found a skilled practitioner and became a regular consumer. I am fortunate to have had the same practitioner for decades; together we have toured my body's battle sites. Some years it was mostly about my neck standing rigid with tension, then the rebellion of my legs, my calves cramping daily from standing for so many hours. During my bout with tendonitis, we coaxed my weakening arms, which hurt to the touch, to not surrender, and then there was the year of the jaw, clenched as if it were the last line of defense as I clamped my way through. These days it's my arthritic hands that are begging for attention. On the table comes relief of pain, a better understanding of how stress manifests, and the means to regulate that stress.

All of this gives me hope that I can find my way back to connection, that my body will someday believe we are safe. I am overdue for a tune-up, and I am tuning in.

○

I am still waiting for the return of my tears. Months after retiring I picked up their signal, as if they were a blip on a radar screen, finally in range after a journey to the most remote place. They are apparently taking the long way home. I documented the day I got that signal in my journal.

In the morning I had listened to a recording of Mary Oliver reading her poem "The Summer Day" as I stared at a doe grazing in our old backyard. I yearned for Mary to be alive, sharing the same world that I was in. I shed a single tear for someone I never met. That evening, I watched *Late Afternoon*, an animated short film about a woman with dementia being served tea by someone she doesn't know—until suddenly she realizes the woman serving her tea is her daughter. They hold each other tight, savoring that fleeting moment of real connection. I remembered my mother-in-law, calling out my name and telling me she loved me during my final visit with her. It was a rare moment of clarity in those last days. At that moment in the film, I cried. Or, rather, my eyes got slightly damp.

Both incidents seem selfish—tears for myself, for my own longing. But maybe that's how it starts, how the dryness of this era ends. Sadness for someone else seems to initiate the conditioned response of my internal professional self: My lacrimal glands clamp off to ensure my helping does not get in the way of my helping.

But I am no longer a professional helper. I want to join the rest of the world in liquid expressions of joy and sadness. I want to connect.

○

I've never been a touchy-feely person, probably because my parents weren't touchy-feely people, yet a few relatives used touch in a controlling way. At a young age I came to associate touch with invasive obligation. I didn't believe I had the right to refuse such touch, and that made me resentful of receiving and giving it.

Touch is used sparingly in the social work profession. This was another sign that I'd chosen the right vocation. Social workers are taught that touch is complicated, which resonates with my experience. Touch might be welcomed, but the receiver also might interpret it as intrusive, disrespectful, or dangerous.

Touching a patient is essential in medical care. Once that boundary is crossed—one stranger touching another—it seems to be assumed that the patient is comfortable with nonessential touching. Nurses understand how powerful touch can be and are not afraid to use it.

I have seen touching mistakes, times when a patient pulled back to avoid a hand on their arm or around their shoulders. But mostly I saw nurses employ profound intuition about when to touch and how, and I saw the tangible ripples of impact in their patients. When we're sick, we're painfully aware of our body's vulnerability. Our body is broken, or we fear it is. Transcending language, touch soothes that fear. Silently it says, *"You're OK, I'm here."*

I watched the nurses touch their patients, and I learned. At first most of my touching was in helping patients when a nurse or tech wasn't there: to get out of their car into a wheelchair to triage, to get out of their bed to the bathroom, to get their shoes on, to eat a meal when they couldn't hold a spoon. I was careful at first, asking a nurse if I should, making sure the patient was steady enough for my inexperienced hands. It wasn't something I had to do, wasn't in my job description, but working in the ER means doing what needs to be done as long as it's safe for the patient.

I saw how nurses touched families who needed support. I put my-self in the position of those family members and often thought if I were that wife or that son, I wouldn't want my hand clasped, my arm tugged gently toward a chair, or a hand that pressed me to sit and re-mained on my shoulder as the doctor shared bad news. Such gestures felt too controlling: *"Come here. Sit. Stay."* But usually, the touch of a nurse wasn't that directive, and even when it was, I couldn't detect any sign of objection from the family member.

With grieving family members, I knew that touch could be part of comfort, a way to ease their pain. I tried it: consciously relaxing my body, opening up my stance, making my hands available, watching for signs that my touch was wanted or welcomed. Often, when I offered a tentative hand on an arm, I'd get wrapped up in a hug.

When the pandemic struck, I saw my elderly mom frequently—delivering her groceries and taking her to medical appointments. Her chronic health problems made her especially vulnerable to Covid. Newly retired, I spent most of the day at home, cleaning out our house for our move. My husband continued to work. Concerned that he could give me the virus and that I might, in turn, infect my mom, he suggested that we limit touching each other as Covid numbers in our city climbed, thinking it would ease in two weeks.

It didn't ease in two weeks, and the absence of touch made Covid even more frightening. I felt more disconnected, more alone. As it be-came clear that this pandemic was going to take a while to play out, we realized that not touching was unsustainable. We continued to take precautions with my mom—we didn't share meals or take her on out-ings, usually visited outside, and were always masked around her—but we soon resumed hugging her because we knew that not being touched worsens fear, loneliness, and feelings of isolation.

Mostly the pandemic made the issue of touching less personally problematic for me. Society's new tentativeness about touch matches my natural ambivalence. I like that we are less likely now to assume someone is comfortable with it, that we hang back a moment to ask, "Are we hugging?"

Before I left the ER, I came to see touch as a tool for connection. It seemed that most people want more touch, even when they don't know you, and especially when they're afraid. Because Covid coincided with my retirement, I had significantly fewer people to interact with. I no longer take touch for granted.

The first line of Ellen Bass's poem "If You Knew" asks, "What if you knew you'd be the last to touch someone?"[3] The poem considers the lives we intersect with on all sorts of levels, never knowing when those people will die and what our touch might mean to them. It's a good reminder in this time of uncertainty. But of course, the timing of life and death is always uncertain.

○

I dream often of the ER. I am not haunted by the nightmare of trauma—rarely do the patients appear. It's the staff I see, usually in our old break room, where we were all thrown together around one table and I learned how to be part of something new, something beyond my age of twenty-eight years.

Because of Covid, once I retired, I couldn't return to visit. I hadn't expected the door to a huge part of my life to close with such finality. I didn't have the resilience of my nurse friend Joan, the nurse and artist who retired and never looked back. I was glad for her. But I needed to see the ER going on without me so I could go on without them. Covid made for a harsh transition.

I got tidbits of updates, the occasional texts from friends who still worked there. I coordinated a delivery of food for all the shifts. I wanted to provide a meal but was told that was harder to manage with staff being so busy. Snacks were preferred, grab-and-go packs of crackers, granola bars, nuts, and fizzy waters. Linda, the supply tech I worked with for about fifteen years, met me at the ER door to unload the items onto a cart she could roll past the locked doors. I hugged her before remembering it was unsafe, later realizing that she might not have appreciated my emotional spontaneity, which surprised me as well.

---

3. Ellen Bass, "If You Knew," in *The Human Line* (Copper Canyon Press, 2007), 50.

I had felt so much fear about the staff's safety and grieved for what they faced every day. I'd been so physically removed from them and their experience that being back there and seeing just one of my old coworkers in person unleashed a torrent of emotion, that old feeling of "this is my team, and they need help." Tears would have burst out and run over my mask if I could cry.

In one recent dream, I see the charge nurse frantically report a lack of rooms and staff. She doesn't have what she needs to provide care for the next bad thing that is coming in right then. The ER staff are overrun and exhausted. I woke up feeling guilty and useless. But I also knew my skill set was not what was needed. They were at war, and I am not that sort of warrior.

In another dream, I walk into that old break room to start my shift and see Joan there, at the table, smiling. Even in the dream I know that Joan is dead.

The reality is that because of Covid, I mourned her alone, isolated from the only people in my life who knew her the way that I did. When she was brought to our ER as a patient with a terminal illness, we were in the renovated space, the new ER where she had never worked. She had nothing to connect to—she did not know us.

In my dream Joan is wearing her scrubs. I tell her I had heard she died. She laughs sheepishly. A medic stands by, red-faced. Apparently, there was some "mistake." My dream self is curious. I have questions but am speechless at my joy in seeing her. She was not one for hugs, so I just gape at her in awe. I hold an edge of the table and crouch down, my face just below hers. I marvel at the wonder of seeing her, of her being in my world again. Still in my dream state, I recall Emma, a medic who had once stood in that break room in my waking life and told me of saving a young woman swept into a flooded culvert. Emma had savored how "incredible it is to have this thing to be so grateful for, a deep-in-your-bones grateful." Emma has also died. I have only this strand of a memory, but it resonates, and in the dream I gaze at a gleeful Joan and feel a deep-in-my-bones grateful.

I have proper tears in that dream. They slide down my cheeks the way they're supposed to, the way they once did long ago. I am free of my self-made constraints. I choke out, "I'm so glad you're alive," hoping these few words are enough to convey all I feel, because they are all I have.

Joan shrugs off my adoration and stands up—it's time to go to work.

Acknowledgments

They're getting it wrong, I think each time I watch the Academy Awards show. The winners' acceptance speeches fill me with anxiety. They start off with thanks to executives and fellow cast and crew members. They take their time, maybe insert some joke or remark about the worthiness of the project, the clock ticking all the while. I pray they will remember there's an orchestra waiting for its cue to swell and thereby mute whatever good intention the winner had to thank their family and loved ones. Those intentions will be silenced, that moment gone forever. It's a grave mistake—putting the people last who mean the most.

I vowed never to do that, as if I'd ever get the chance. I am not on that stage, and I haven't been awarded anything, but the lesson applies. I begin with those the least involved in this project but who have paid the highest cost of knowing me—my family: I couldn't have written this without you.

My time in the ER didn't just change who I was as a person and a social worker; it changed who I was as a wife, mother, and daughter. I once thought that I succeeded at keeping those changes hidden, as if my compartmentalization acted as alchemy, providing me with an alternate identity to embody, but now I know better.

My husband decided long ago that it's better for him (and presumably us) to not read my work prior to publishing. Despite knowing little of what I write before it's out in the world, too late to be reeled back in, he supports me unconditionally—my right to say what I want to say the way that I want to say it. That is a disturbing amount of trust, and I hope I deserve it.

Thanks to my kids for their love and support, for being patient with my limitations and coping mechanisms, and for giving me perspective through having lives and interests far beyond my world of worst-case scenarios.

Thank you to my parents for raising me to have my own opinions and for stretching to understand and support me.

To my friends, who, unlike my family, I didn't even try to protect. Instead, I depended on you, recklessly subjecting you to stories and using you as my demarcation line of just how far I strayed from normal. You listened. You didn't judge me, and you kept humor in my life. With you I could step outside of my roles of social worker, wife, and mother.

To Katherine Cerulean, my writing-critique partner who quickly became a close friend many years ago, thank you for being beside me, chapter by chapter. I invited you into a hellish landscape, and you stepped in fearlessly. On our journey you brought along your insight, guidance, and legendary relentless cheer. So much of this book bears your careful consideration and steady influence.

To Denise Lockamy, my RN friend who read the entire manuscript early on and said indeed it did make sense and was worth reading. You were one of only a few people who could truthfully say, "Yes, that happened. Yes, it was like that." Thanks also for supplying details I'd left out, including the comical adventures of "Tweed."

Karen Kassinger, you came into the project in its later phase and supplied the desperately needed energy and contacts to push me toward the finish line. Your deep sharing about touch from a nurse's perspective influenced my writing, and your support and belief in this work steadied me in storms of self-doubt. Deep bow.

To Mary Overton and Mark All for reading chapters and providing suggestions and support—thank you.

Thank you to Janisse Ray for gifting me with selected chapter edits and the support that gave me the confidence to continue.

I am grateful to several editors, with their endless patience and excellent eyes. Lee Ann Pingel, with Expert Eye Editing, waded in on an early draft, learning my inner language, becoming the interpreter of me to me. Then Gail Karwoski, Katherine Richards, and Jaye Whitney Debber, all working with Girl Friday Books, worked their magic with tenacious insight. Thank you all for making the book better at every step.

And finally, to the entire team at Girl Friday Books, especially Abi Pollokoff, who guided me through the process with skill and kindness.

Now, cue the orchestra and I'll make my exit.

Bibliography

Abram, David. *Becoming Animal*. Vintage Books, 2011.

American Psychiatric Association. *Desk Reference to the Diagnostic Criteria from DSM-5*. American Psychiatric Publishing, 2013.

Augsburger, David. *Caring Enough to Hear and Be Heard*. Baker Publishing Group, 1982.

Bass, Ellen. "If You Knew," in *The Human Line*. Copper Canyon Press, 2007.

Bechdel, Alison. *The Secret to Superhuman Strength*. Mariner Books, 2021.

Bride, Brian E., Margaret M. Robinson, Bonnie Yegidis, and Charles R. Figley. "Development and Validation of the Secondary Traumatic Stress Scale." *Research on Social Work Practice* 14, no. 1 (2004): 27–35. https://doi.org/10.1177/1049731503254106.

Campbell, Joseph, with Bill Moyers. *The Power of Myth*. Doubleday, 1988.

The Commonwealth Fund. "Women in the U.S. More Likely to Die in Pregnancy, Childbirth, and Postpartum Than Women in Other High-Income Nations." Released November 18, 2020. https://www.commonwealthfund.org/press-release/2020/women-us-more-likely-die-pregnancy-childbirth-and-postpartum-women-other-high.

Dana, Deb. *Anchored: How to Befriend Your Nervous System Using Polyvagal Theory*. Sounds True, 2021.

Degeest, Sofie, Hannah Keppler, and Paul Corthals. "The Effect of Age on Listening Effort." *Journal of Speech, Language, and Hearing Research* 58, no. 5 (2015): 1592–1600. https://doi.org/10.1044/2015_JSLHR-H-14-0288.

Epstein, Mark. *The Trauma of Everyday Life*. Penguin Books, 2014.

Erikson, Erik. *Childhood and Society*. W. W. Norton & Company, 1993.

Erikson, Erik. *Identity and the Life Cycle*. W. W. Norton & Company, 1994.

Gentry, J. Eric, Anna B. Baranowsky, and Kathleen Dunning, "The Accelerated Recovery Program (ARP) for Compassion Fatigue," in *Treating Compassion Fatigue*, ed. Charles R. Figley. Brunner-Routledge, 2002.

Harper, Faith. *This Is Your Brain on Anxiety: What Happens and What Helps*. Microcosm Publishing, 2018.

Joinson, Carla. "Coping with Compassion Fatigue." *Nursing* 22, no. 4 (1992): 116, 118–120.

Josselson, Ruthellen. *Paths to Fulfillment*. Oxford University Press, 2017.

Jung, Carl G. "Synchronicity: An Acausal Connecting Principle." Translated by R. F. C. Hull. In *The Collected Works of C. G. Jung, Volume 8*, edited by In H. Read, M. Fordham, & G. Adler. Princeton University Press, 1973. http://naqiao.hk/libros_fortea /synchronicity_an_acausal_connecting_principlp-CG_Jung.pdf.

Malesic, Jonathan. "How Men Burn Out." *New York Times*, January 4, 2022. https://www.nytimes.com/2022/01/04/opinion/burnout -men-signs.html.

March of Dimes. "Nowhere to Go: Maternity Care Deserts Across the US." Accessed 2024. https://marchofdimes.org/maternity-care -deserts-report.

Maslach, Christina, Wilmar B. Schaufeli, and Michael P. Leiter. "Job Burnout." *Annual Review of Psychology*, 52 (2001): 397–422. https://doi.org/10.1146/annurev.psych.52.1.397.

Meier, Barbara. "Jerry Garcia Speaks with Barbara Meier." *Tricycle: The Buddhist Review*, Spring 1992. https://tricycle.org/magazine /jerry-garcia-speaks-with-barbara-meier/.

Oleksy, Ernest M. "A Brief Review of Freudian and Jungian Theories." *The Downtown Review* 5, no. 2 (2019): https://engagedscholarship .csuohio.edu/tdr/vol5/iss2/4.

Piaget, Jean. *The Construction of Reality in the Child*. Translated by M. Cook. Basic Books, 1954.

Salzberg, Sharon. *Real Change: Mindfulness to Heal Ourselves and the World*. Flatiron Books, 2020.

San Diego State University. "Secondary Stress Scale." https://theacademy.sdsu.edu/wp-content/uploads/2019/09/STSSwithscoreinterpretation.pdf.

Shafir, Rebecca. *The Zen of Listening*. Quest Books, 2000.

Tolle, Eckhart. *A New Earth*. Plume Books, 2006.

Vogler, Christopher. *The Writer's Journey*. 3rd ed. Michael Wiese Productions, 2007.

Winnicott, D. W. *Playing and Reality*. Tavistock Publications, 1971.

About the Author

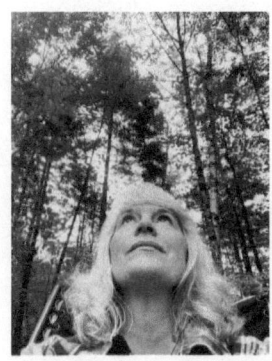 KATHRYN KYKER spent twenty-nine years as a social worker in the ER, rising from the role of patient advocate to social work manager, where she created a case management program and supervised a team of patient advocates. A licensed MSW, she received her bachelor's degree in social work from Western Carolina University and a master's degree in social work from the University of Georgia. Kathryn received her hospital's Emergency Medical Service Special Achievement Award in 2008 for significant support of outreach efforts by EMTs and paramedics to help frequent users of emergency services.

Kathryn's writing has appeared in publications such as *Salvation South*, *Boom Magazine*, and *Flagpole*. She's had two short films produced from her screenplays. She now spends her time writing and biking with her husband in Georgia and North Carolina and curates a summer film series sponsored by the Osher Lifelong Learning Institute at the University of Georgia.

www.ingramcontent.com/pod-product-compliance
Lightning Source LLC
Chambersburg PA
CBHW021712120626
46545CB00004B/1529